Raw Success

The Key to *100% Raw Vegan Longevity*

Matthew J. Monarch

Edited by: Michelle Sabathné

Layout & Design: Liz Johnson
Cover Concept: Desire'e Martinez
Proofreading: Angela Stokes

Library of Congress Catalog Card Number on file:
ISBN # 978-0-9795701-0-0
Copyright ©2007 by Matt Monarch
First Edition, September 2007

Monarch Publishing Company
12709 Byron Ave.,
Granada Hills, CA 91344
USA

Disclaimer:
The following information is for education only and is not
meant to diagnose, prescribe, or treat illness. It is valuable to
seek the guidance of an alternative health care professional
before making any changes to one's diet and lifestyle.

DEDICATION

I often dream about what it would be like to meet those Raw Pioneers who have passed on, for whom I have great admiration. Imagining the numerous questions that would ramble out of my mouth upon meeting them, I realize how blessed I am to have Dr. Fred Bisci as a mentor. Fred always provides accurate, scientific explanations for the experiences, discoveries, and unfavorable results of many well-respected Health Pioneers. (Often Fred's explanations for these patterns seem to not be understood even by those having these experiences.)

I dedicate *Raw Success* to Dr. Fred Bisci. I have met no other man who has impacted this planet in such a miraculous way. Fred's relationship with God and connection to Spirit is, I feel, without a doubt the main reason why he understands these "unknown" health concepts so well and has such a high success rate with his patients.

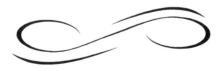

A WORD FROM THE AUTHOR

Science is suspicious of our eating habits, society gawks, families fret, and doctors shake their red faces – it is clear that as Raw Foodists we are mostly on our own, and must learn from each other.

There are controversial issues discussed in this book. My sole desire is to be of service, and this gives me courage to go way outside the lines.

The section I am most delighted to share in Raw Success is entitled, *The Science Behind It All*, which can be found in the middle of the book on the glossy pages. The information in this section has the potential to shift human consciousness and the way medicine is practiced today. While reading *Raw Success*, you may wish to frequently reference *The Science Behind It All* for an even deeper understanding of the concepts presented throughout the book.

It is my intention that this book serves as a complete guide to your *Raw Success*. For those just beginning, who are perhaps not so familiar with my work, I recommend first reading Appendix A, *'What You Don't Eat'*, which outlines simple steps for transitioning to a healthy Raw Lifestyle.

My hope is that these pages herein add decades of vital living for both the person new to the Raw Adventure, as well as for the Raw Food Pioneers who wish to continue their journey with optimal long-term success.

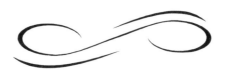

CONTENTS

INTRODUCTION
Interrogating the Raw Diet

Most of us go RAW to enjoy the full potential of our body – energy, joy and beauty, throughout a long and pain free existence. Sounds Heavenly. Yet as I look around the Raw community a few questions emerge:

> *Is the Raw Lifestyle making good on its promise for long life and health?*
> *Where are all the amazingly vital Raw Foodists, living past 100?*
> *Why aren't Raw Food Eaters living decades longer than cooked food eaters?*

If you look at the Raw Pioneers – Paul Bragg, Herbert Shelton, Bernard Jensen, William Esser, Johnny Lovewisdom – they lived between 80 and 93 years, or less. It seems to me that a 100% Raw Food Eater does amazingly well in the beginning, compared to a cooked food eater. Diseases are healed, persistent pounds are shed, and depressions lift. However, as we continue eating Raw, over time, we lose our advantage and the gap closes. *Raw Success* addresses why the Raw Foodist is not thriving well past the age of 100, and reveals how we can encourage ceaseless regeneration.

My Story

Seven years ago, my world went from hamburgers to celery. Overnight, I become a 100% Raw Foodist. One single word describes my experience: transformation – *rapid* transformation. I rejuvenated, became younger, experienced electric vitality, and for the first time ever, my life took on an undeniable spiritual dimension. Convinced of the benefits of Raw Living, I wanted to progress quickly.

After my sixth year of consuming exclusively Raw Food, the tides of transformation changed direction. In fact, my body stopped becoming younger. This body that was so thrilled to throw off years of stored toxins and waste, had caught up to the present day, and I *started to age on a Raw Diet.* Aging was inevitable and had to happen at some point, but I became extremely interested in ways to delay aging and increase vitality, for as long as possible.

Everything I have learned – from myself, books, "experts", the bruises of experience and all the triumphs of experimentation – I offer to you here, for your long-term Raw Success.

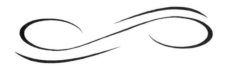

1
LIVING FOREVER
The Fountain of Youth

There are many reasons to eat only Raw Foods. Not the least of which is the reversal of time – to become younger, to once again experience the beauty, health, and vibrancy of youth.

Why do we become younger with a Raw Lifestyle?
The answer is simple:
We eat less food.

It's true. Profoundly and simply – *the key to becoming younger is eating less food.* The body jumps at any chance to heal itself and become younger. Eating less food gives our body the ideal opportunity it's been waiting for! Compared to cooked and/or processed food, Raw Food is "less food" in two ways: *Less Quantity* and *Better Quality.*

1. *Quantity:* Eating less bulk – while Raw Food is nutrient dense, it is mostly just water, and thus, *actual* bulk is less than concentrated cooked foods. We get the nutrients we need without having to Super Size.

2. *Quality:* Eating better quality food – cooking and processing not only deplete the nutrients in food, in some cases it also mutates the cellular struc-

ture of the elements composing that food. These mutations are often harmful to the body, whereas organic live foods are harmless and mostly water: water distilled by nature.

Obstruction-Free

Did you know that the human body is a Perfectionist? The body's dream come true would be for us to live in a pristine environment on water alone, breathing in the heavenly fragrance of pure clean air. I am not going to explain in detail the theory about how and why Breatharianism is possible; that's another book in itself. (While I have not experienced this myself, there are reports of numerous humans on this planet who live and **thrive on air, water and sunshine** ONLY.) In truth, everything else is obstructive to the body to one degree or another. An *obstruction* is anything that hinders one's progress towards optimal health. In other words, if we are not Breatharians living off pure pristine water and air, then we are putting obstructive elements in our system.

The real question is:
Which foods are least obstructive?
Raw Foods

Another way of saying 'least obstructive' is 'least damaging'. Raw Food can be considered an obstructive element to our body, but it is much, much less damaging than cooked food. When we eat this nutrient-rich Raw Food, made of mostly water, there are fewer obstructive elements entering our system than if we were to consume large portions of dense dead food made with ingredients we can't pronounce.

Similarly, someone eating an Intermediate Diet, which eliminates refined sugars and processed starches is putting fewer obstructive elements into their body compared to someone on the Standard American Diet.

The Reward

*Eating **less obstructive food** frees up the body's energy to **detoxify** itself of anything anti-life that may be stored in its cells and tissues.*

Also, if you are eating only Raw Foods and drinking their juices, you get the added bonus of rapid regeneration of your cells, tissues, organs, and blood, all the while furnishing the body with the finest nourishment for continued smooth performance and well-being.

To become younger is to experience *massive regeneration*, so that one not only heals the typical damage that cells experience during the course of a single day, but the body also has enough surplus energy to repair long-term damage sustained from our past habits as well. The results are that we look and feel renewed. Add to that a rich spiritual connectedness, which is a natural part of being Raw, and it is like Heaven right here on Earth. If you had your wish, wouldn't you want to become younger forever, reaching higher and higher levels of vitality and health?

There comes a point, however, after the body has thrown off its major load of toxins and has healed to a considerable degree, that the process of becoming younger stops and aging begins. It was during my mid-20s that I crossed over to a Raw Lifestyle. By year six, I had already released most of my worst toxicity and that's when I stopped becoming younger. Taking youthfulness to the next level would require one to eat less food, but as you will learn, that decision can have surprisingly negative consequences on our lifespan.

The Observation

The effects of Raw Living have fascinated me since I began to learn about this lifestyle. I began to watch in hopes of learning from their experiences. Often, I would meet men and women who started their Raw journey much later in life than me. I began to notice something strange. Their process of becoming younger showed no signs of slowing, even after 10-15 years Raw – they were still healing, becoming more energized and more beautiful.[1]

I discovered that the reason was this: They had more damage and toxins to clean up from the added years of poor living, so they were enjoying a longer process of becoming younger.

To illustrate this fact, there is a story I want to share with you, and it requires a brief introduction to a great man. Dr. Fred Bisci has been my primary mentor during this Raw journey. He has a PhD in Nutrition, and has seen well over 25,000 people during his 50-year career. Because of Dr. Bisci's extremely high success rate for helping heal people from degenerative disease, he is quite respected and sought out by those who suffer. In addition, Fred has been Raw over four decades. There

---

[1] The elders who transition to a 100% Raw Diet seem to stand out far more fully and vibrantly in contrast to others in their age range. It is really quite extraordinary to see.

is a priceless interview with him in my first book, *Raw Spirit*.

Now, onto the story:

Dr. Fred Bisci's mom had a stroke at age 84, and her doctors told her she had only a few months to live. Fred convinced his mom to improve her diet under his guidance and his sister's supervision. She recovered swiftly and lived to the ripe old age of 101! Her process of becoming younger lasted longer than mine. Already at death's door, the only place to go was UP! Fred's mom was given so much extra life and energy because there was a huge amount of cleaning to be done. Not only did she evade death for quite some time, but she also pushed on to live years past many of our Raw Pioneers.

The Law of Adaptation

How did we get clogged up in the first place?
The body adapts to what we do OR do not do.

As was highlighted previously, one of the main reasons why a Raw Lifestyle makes us feel and become younger is the results of the detox that takes place with an improved diet.

It is crucial to understand the adaptation ability of our bodies. As many of us know from personal experience, the cleaner our diet, the more sensitive we become. For example, if someone completely eliminates processed starches and greasy foods from their diet, but three years later eats a slice of pizza, they will inevitably feel ill. *The body adapts to what we do or do not do.* When we improve our diet, we can no longer tolerate certain lower quality foods.

If you were to ingest an entire tablespoon of arsenic, chances are high that you would die. However, if you were to take a drop of arsenic once every three days and very gradually over many months increase the dosage, after three years you could likely survive that same tablespoon of arsenic. Building up your arsenic tolerance is not the healthiest thing to do for long-term health, but the example illustrates the amazing adaptive response of our bodies.

Not far removed from the arsenic example, is what most of us have been doing all our lives. Imagine feeding a newborn baby a Quarter Pounder® with cheese. Your insides may shout in protest to the idea – "No, don't you dare!" The results could be devastating, similar perhaps to us suddenly consuming an entire tablespoon of arsenic.

We clearly see the mistake it would be to feed greasy fast food to an infant. What we may not be so quick to realize is that many children are given a version of fast food, being fed processed baby food three times a day. The constant runny nose warning is eventually silenced by repetition. Years pass, a variety of cooked/processed foods are added little by little, until eventually they can tackle that juicy hamburger. Building up your tolerance to "plastic food" is not the healthiest thing to do for long-term health, but you can do it – *you did it*.

As a 100% Raw Food Eater, you become pure and clean again, *like a newborn*. The longer you are Raw, the more sensitive you become. Processed foods you ate before are no longer tolerated. I have been on a Raw Diet for almost seven years. I am convinced that half a hamburger would put me in the hospital. If you were to give Dr. Fred Bisci, 40-year Raw Foodist, the same half hamburger, it could end in disaster. Yet most people on the planet can eat two hamburgers, slap their knee and say "Mmmmm".

{The glossy section in the middle of the book, "The Science Behind It All," explains exactly what happens on a cellular level as the body "adapts" and why we become more sensitive.}

Air Quality

It is essential to talk about the concept of air quality. *Air is another food we ingest.* The quality of our air has a significant impact on the quality of our health.

The bodies of those starting a Raw Lifestyle in their late 40s/early 50s, have greater resistance to a toxic environment. Compared to them, I have considerably less tolerance for pollutants. For example, in a smoky room I am coughing and headachy, while they may show no signs of discomfort. Obviously, my clean young body is more susceptible. On a cellular level I do not have as much buffer against car fumes, smoky rooms, detergents and chemicals.

Bottom line: Toxins have a more damaging effect on a cleaner body.

Exposure to these toxins will not shorten our life in the long-run. As healthy eaters, we rapidly heal from the damage done and will live a healthier, longer life if doing the 100% Raw Diet correctly.

However, if I were forced to live *day and night* in a smoky room with a 55-year-old man who had been Raw five years, and a man on a Standard American Diet, my seven-year Raw, early 30s body would suffer the most damage. The 55-year-old five year Raw Foodist would sustain minor cellular injury, and the SAD dieter may never feel a thing. Without new, good quality air and an opportunity to regenerate, my higher level of health would actually work against me in this situation.

Which brings us to this ironic fact:

A body that is not full of vitality, and is in a weakened state, can endure and live longer under adverse conditions than a cleaner body. *{Please note: This statement does not say that a less-vital body will "thrive and experience amazing vitality", it merely implies survival.}*

To illustrate this hypothesis, Hilton Hotema offers the perfect example in his book, *Man's Higher Consciousness.*

In a clinical experiment, a group of scientists put Bird-A in a glass cage with no air outlets. Breath by breath, the bird exhaled CO_2, and the air in the cage became increasingly more toxic. Because the process happened gradually, the bird was able to adapt to the CO_2 rich environment. Bird-A was then removed from the glass cage. Bird-B was placed in the same CO_2 rich environment. Bird-B died in moments from shock. Bird-B had no time to adapt like Bird-A, and the sudden extreme toxicity made it impossible to sustain life.

In addition to foods, we are very sensitive to air quality,

to the toxic load we breathe with each inhale. Based on the bird example above, it stands to reason that if you took a man who walked this pristine Earth 5000 years ago and dropped him into the current polluted state of our planet, most likely he would not survive long.

Raw Food Makes Us More Sensitive

It is undeniable: I am dramatically more sensitive to cigarette smoke now as a Raw Foodist than when my diet was cooked. The damage to my cleaner, vulnerable cells is evident. In my first book, *Raw Spirit*, I wrote about a Raw woman who smokes cigarettes. She was unaware how injurious smoking was for her compared to someone on a typical diet. I encouraged her to either quit smoking or start eating cooked food, because the cleaner our diet, the more harmful foreign substances are to our body.

Is it true to say that a cooked, processed food eater lives as long as the Raw Foodist because they can better endure the present condition on Earth? Does the Raw Foodist age and die prematurely, compared to their potential of 100+ years, because of our environment?

I feel that the toxic environment is one of the main reasons the gap narrows in the long-run, and cooked and Raw Food Eaters die at the same age. Luckily, there is a solution, which I will describe in detail, along with the other reasons why we do not seem to be succeeding in the long-run. If done correctly, the 100% Raw

Food Diet is the ultimate diet for the human organism, giving us the ability to thrive well beyond the century mark. More than anything, your body wants these natural "miracles" to take place.

The Young Raw Foodist

Someone who starts young and stays Raw reaches a point of extreme cleanliness early. After a few years they have already cleansed, regenerated, and become younger. The body quickly repairs a large portion of the damage done from the previous years of processed foods and substances. Additionally, they can cleanse deeper on a cellular level compared to someone who started later in life (like Fred's mom) making them even more sensitive. At this level of immaculate inner health, the long-term Raw Food Eater is more susceptible to our Earth's polluted environment, and toxic chemicals.

It seems as if it is more advisable to become Raw
at age 40 versus age 20.
Is there a way around this?
Yes, with Consistency, Cleansing and
The Optimal Diet.
{By the end of the book, this answer will be
fully clear to you.}

2
STABILIZING OUT
Quality and Quantity

If you become Raw at age 25, in less than a decade, there is a great chance that your body will stabilize and start to age instead of becoming younger.

Let's look closer at why this forecast for the long-term Raw Foodist is seemingly inevitable. Knowing "why" will help us discover how to go in a different direction.

In Chapter 1 we said that becoming younger happens when we *eat less food*. Once again, the magical combination Raw Food offers is *better quality* (nutrient rich) meals and *less quantity* of food.

Many Raw Foodists come from a SAD or processed diet background. Raw Food is the highest *quality* you can ingest, taxing our bodies the least. The chemical elements of a baked potato or hamburger are damaging to our bodies, whereas live Raw Foods are perfectly made to nourish and energize the body. Furthermore, Raw Food is mostly water! Although the meals you eat may look similar in size compared to your previously cooked menu, if you were to blend a large Raw salad to liquid, and then remove the water content by placing it in a dehydrator or oven for a few hours, you would be left with a mere handful of powder. Thus, the actual bulk of food eaten in a Raw Meal is considerably less than a cooked food meal – addressing the factor of *quantity*. Higher quality food and smaller meals are less obstructive, making them the perfect recipe for regeneration.

Less Food Can Lead To No Food

Based on the age you begin a Raw Diet, your health condition, and your consistency with eating the same quantity and quality of food each day, over time your body will *stabilize out*. The massive detox stops, and then at some point you start to age because you've caught up to your own evolution. The only way to restart the process of becoming younger is to *eat less food*. You would need to eat less and less over the years to continue the process of age reversal. This is futile – all Raw Foodists would eventually be eating miniscule amounts of food or become Liquidarian, living exclusively on liquid. Then what?

The benefits of extreme dieting would indeed include slower aging, increased strength, vitality, and phenomenal spiritual receptivity. However, exponentially more sensitive than a Raw Foodist, a long-term Liquidarian has even less endurance for adverse conditions and their longevity would be compromised in the long-run, not from diet, but from toxins in the air they breathe.

What Is "Normal" To You?

Our body is the most ready and willing servant for our happiness. It is always pushing us towards greater levels of perfection and health. Whenever it is given a chance through fasting or improved diet, the body goes into immediate healing.

In an ideal, pristine environment, our body could live on pure water, small amounts of food and nutrient dense, flowery, fragrant air. Yet we are not dwelling on a "Garden of Eden" planet anymore. As crazy as it might sound, we actually need to stop the body from loving us too well and pushing us too far forward.

Let me explain.

There is a new concept I'd like to introduce to you. To describe this new idea, I've coined the term: *Stabilizing Out.*

Stabilizing Out happens when the body gets accustomed to a habitual quantity and a certain quality of food. Biologically, we stabilize out, no matter what our diet is like – whether we are on a cooked diet eating three fast food meals a day, or a Raw Diet eating two small meals a day. If we are consistent, eventually, our body settles into a "normal" food day; this is called "stabilizing out".

Once you *stabilize out,* eating more than your usual amount of food often results in a feeling of illness or fatigue. Furthermore, because the body loves progress, even if you are "perfect" and eat exact daily portions, at some point, your body will again try to raise the bar by encouraging you to eat less food. Often this nudge towards progress will be felt as sluggishness after eating your typical meal. This is the body encouraging a reduced appetite, so that you can reach higher levels of health and energy.

Unless your diet continues to improve, at some point you will suffer sluggishness and begin to age. The danger is that the cleaner your diet, the faster this progression occurs, and the more sensitive you become to adverse environmental conditions as the years go on.

Giving In

To avoid discomfort and regain vitality, many give in to the body's prodding and eat smaller meals. Can you see how this process is never ending? The body is always moving toward greater levels of optimal health, becoming cleaner and more efficient, needing less to thrive. This applies no matter where you are starting.

For example, a long-term Liquidarian who has stabilized out in a routine of 4 veggie and/or fruit juices a day, would experience lowered energy and physical discomfort if they were to drink a 5th or 6th glass of juice. JUICE! What's more, their body will eventually encourage them to drink 3½ glasses of juice rather than their typical 4. At some point they will feel discomfort and sluggishness unless they reduce their juice intake.

Before becoming Raw, I ate three processed food meals a day — mostly microwave chicken patties, Subway sandwiches, In-and-Out Burger — the diet of a college bachelor. My body tolerated the menu well; I exercised, rarely overate, and felt energized. As a Raw Foodist, I thrive on much less. For years now I have consistently eaten two simple Raw Meals a day. My body has *stabilized out*. If I consume larger portions or more than two meals, immediately my energy drops. Additionally, my body is now trying to push me further by creating occasional bouts of sluggishness after a typical sized meal. It's saying, "Eat less fat and sugar". What's incredible is that 99% of the human population would feel extremely hungry and energized on my diet, yet my body wants to keep moving forward, into less and less food intake.

Will I Get Enough Nutrients if I'm Eating Less Food?

The nutritional needs of each individual vary depending on your level of cellular cleanliness. The more you detox, the cleaner you become on a cellular level. As you stabilize out at new healthier levels of eating, you will have more energy and need less food.

The person eating a Standard American Diet requires more calories and nutrients to function well. The person eating an all-Raw Diet can accomplish the same endurance with less food because when the body is clean, it is more efficient and requires less fuel for energy. Someone who has been on a Raw Diet 40 years will need less food than someone who has been eating Raw for only five years. And a 5-year Raw Foodist needs less food than someone eating Raw for 1 year.

{I recommend reading the section entitled "The Science Behind It All", which explains exactly what happens on a cellular level as the body evolves to new levels of health.}

Squeaky Clean

Many start the Raw Lifestyle to reach "ultimate health". Naturally there are some who wish to become as pure as possible in their Raw choices, excluding certain foods or combinations that feel too dense or not ideal. I personally do not recommend eliminating concentrated foods such as nuts and seeds. I want to comment further about this issue, as it is becoming quite popular with some Raw Foodists.

Some people think that eliminating concentrated foods such as nuts is a dietary improvement because the digestive system is less taxed, thereby bringing us closer to an optimal state. This is a half-truth. Many years ago, when the Earth's environment was pure and pristine, eliminating concentrated foods would have been beneficial. If done correctly, the body becomes more vital, strong, and in tune to heightened spiritual experiences. However, in today's compromised air quality, by cutting out nuts, one would ultimately shorten their lifespan because of their vulnerability to the current adverse conditions facing our planet.

In the long-run, eliminating concentrated foods lowers our endurance for adverse conditions, and any inconsistent actions in the future will take a greater toll on our vitality. Why walk on a tight rope? Not only do I feel there are immense benefits from the nutrients nuts and seeds provide, but they also help to slow our body's evolution.

Too clean: We do not want to become so pure that the environment takes its toll on us in the long-run. For 99% of the Raw Foodists reading this book, your diet is not in a danger zone. It takes many decades on a consistent, "extreme" Raw Diet before you need be concerned about the environment's effect unless you are living in an extremely toxic environment. However, it's good to be aware of factors that play a part in our long-term Raw Success. *{There are other reasons why 95% of Raw Foodists do not succeed in the long-run, which I will continue to share with you later in this book.}*

Super Sensitivity

Even after a mere five day fast, my body threatens to evolve. Returning to my regular meals is a great adjustment and I usually experience grogginess as my body makes room for the unwanted quantity of food. My body is shocked to be eating again, and that is after only five days of abstinence! Imagine eating very little food for decades... Consistency would be crucial to avoid shocking your system.

In my previous book *Raw Spirit*, I wrote about a man who only ate 12oz of food once a day for many years. A friend convinced him to try 16oz in his daily meal. That extra four ounces almost killed him. We each have a threshold. Like I said before, if I were to eat half a hamburger today, there is a great chance I would need medical attention. After seven years on a 100% Raw Diet, I can no longer tolerate what used to be a daily ritual. In contrast, the majority of folks can eat two thick-meat hamburgers, and feel fine. Again, it is extremely beneficial to understand that if you were to feed 45-year Raw Veteran, Dr. Fred Bisci, the same half hamburger you gave me, he would likely suffer some potentially lethal consequences.

As the above example illustrates, the further you take your diet by eating less quantity and higher quality food, the more sensitive you become to inconsistencies. A Liquidarian will not only be more sensitive to the current condition of Earth, but there is a greater chance of shocking their system from any change to their typical diet.

It is difficult to convey the sensitivity issue of extreme long-term dieting. Most people don't experience this type of danger because they never take their eating to that level. Even as 100% Raw Foodists, we cannot truly fathom the sensitivity of a Liquidarian or Breatharian.

There are many layers of sensitivity. One who consumes rich Raw Food dishes frequently during the day, would experience a much greater sensitivity in the long-run if they were to *consistently* eat only two light Raw Meals a day. The lighter the food, and the more the body is allowed to "fast" with an empty stomach, sensitivity levels drastically increase.

I believe that many of the Raw Pioneers who didn't live past the century mark ran into health complications because they did not do the 100% Raw Food Diet optimally. At some point their bodies may have reached a level of crisis. Confused, they may have returned to eating animal protein or other cooked foods, attempting to remedy the problem. This type of shock to their system could have ended in disaster.

Having read what I've written so far, please, do not be scared of becoming too sensitive. It is something to be aware of for *long-term* success so that we can adjust accordingly. This book is going to guide you to your longest possible lifespan, potentially far surpassing the century mark on the 100% Raw Food Diet.

To Summarize

In summary, there are two main factors to consider:

1. *Consistency*
If you have been consistent for quite awhile in quality and/or quantity of food, your body has stabilized to a new level of health. Once stable on a Raw Diet,

we must be cautious with our *quality* and *quantity* of food. It is unwise to yo-yo between cooked and Raw Food Diets. The longer you have been doing this, the more sensitive you become. Any changes you make are best done gradually, to avoid bodily shock.

2. *Being "too dirty" or "too clean"*

We do not want to suffer the bodily harm, lack of vitality, and disease from a processed, cooked or SAD diet. Neither do we want to get boxed into eating only very small, basic Raw Meals or a liquid diet. That level of cleanliness would make us very susceptible to our environment.

Raw Foods are powerful - they are a fire, not a feather. It is in our best interest to go deep in our education about the Raw Lifestyle, so that we can make wise choices now and in the future. The trick is to keep moving forward with the least detrimental effect to us now and in the long-run.

3
OPTIMAL LIFESTYLE

How can I become more balanced?
Not too much; not too little; just right.

The Balance Beam of Longevity

There are three main elements that need to be in balance for optimal longevity:

1. The food and/or substances we intake
2. Our external environment
3. Cleansing *{which we'll focus on in the next few chapters}*

Naturally, a long happy life also involves mental, emotional and spiritual health, but let's focus on the physical realm for the moment.

We can think of longevity as if we are walking on a balance beam – we desire the perfect *quality* and *amount* of food, so that we can put the aging process into slow motion, yet avoid becoming so clean that we suffer harm from our environment. As illustrated in the following diagrams, the ideal diet is healthy, yet not too extreme, giving us a sturdy endurance in the midst of our atmosphere. The purpose of *Raw Success* is to guide you along the optimal path, leading you far beyond what was ever imagined possible for your energy and your life, for decades to come.

Environment Shortens Life

Diet Is Too Clean
- - - - - - - - - - - - -

Not Enough Food

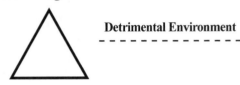

Detrimental Environment
- - - - - - - - - - - - - -

When we continually improve our diet, the body evolves to higher and higher levels of cleanliness. If our "diet is too clean" in quality and quantity, in the long-run, our body's refined sensitivity becomes vulnerable to the toxic everyday environment.

This state of purity is like plush white carpet that no one wants to put in the house because it will show every speck of dirt. Living in this rather filthy 21st Century world, you track in grime from outside all the time. I am not suggesting that you tar and pave your body to withstand the Indy 500 coming through (as is the case with most SAD Dieters), but it is wise to have a buffer.

Food Shortens Life

Environment Not A Danger
- - - - - - - - - - - - - - -

Too Much Food

Detrimental Diet
- - - - - - - - - - - -

Poor quality cooked or processed foods, substances like drugs and alcohol, or consistent stressful eating habits like overeating, snacking and late night meals (even the best quality foods), can also shorten life. Then the greatest threat to long life is not environment, it is diet.

Longest Duration Of Life

Optimal Diet   **Environment Least Detrimental**

‑ ‑ ‑ ‑ ‑ ‑ ‑ ‑ ‑ ‑ ‑ ‑ ‑ **Optimal Food Intake** ‑ ‑ ‑ ‑ ‑ ‑ ‑ ‑ ‑ ‑ ‑ ‑ ‑

As in all things of wisdom, balance is the key. When we can eat sufficiently for our needs and not let our body's evolution get ahead of our planet's environmental evolution, then we achieve the greatest possible longevity. A proposed "Optimal Food Intake" will be revealed in Chapter 9.

The "New Environment"

Did you know that we are essentially aliens in our own environment? It can be an experience of profound shock and tremendous grief for us to fully realize that Planet Earth 2007 has become overloaded with harmful toxins compared to Mother Earth 3000 BC. The air we breathe is saturated with waste and every molecule has grime in it. Undeniably, we are not breathing fresh air anymore; we are inhaling a *new environment*.

Imagine you were swimming through the air. Yet instead of clean translucent aqua, the "water" you are swimming in is brown. Just as the bird could exist in its CO_2 glass cage, and just as fish are adapting to survive in our polluted rivers and streams, we have managed to adapt to our world. The "murky water" has become part of our beings. Fortunately, our body has the ability to adjust, if the process is gradual and not overly shocking. The problem is that this happens at the expense of our health and longevity.

The cleaner we become, the less endurance we have for toxins – dietary or environmental. You may be thinking that the only way to avoid this mess is to seek solace somewhere like the pristine Himalayan Mountains (relative to the rest of the planet, this land is uncontaminated and the air is refreshingly clean), eventually needing to eat little or no food, spending your days in the highs of physical and spiritual existence. That is an option, which would indeed increase your lifespan, yet it may not be the most practical for you and your family.

Although improbable for most, let's entertain the Himalayan option for the sake of further understanding.

Pristine Living For Even Greater Health And Longevity

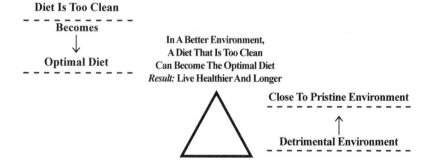

With pristine air quality, the diagram for optimal longevity looks a little different. This pristine environment does not threaten our body now or in the long-run. Because we do not have to protect ourselves from a Detrimental Environment, we can eat less food. If we were previously eating a diet that was "Too Clean" for the Detrimental Environment we lived in, it would now be just right (the Optimal Diet) in a pristine environment. Why is this significant? Because the fewer obstructing {damaging} foods we put in our body, while staying in balance with our environment, the less we age, thereby continuing to progress in health and ultimately lengthen our life.

Moving Backwards

There is a drawback to pristine living. If, after years of living in pure air, you decided to return to your old "dirty" environment for any reason, such as a family emergency, your endurance for adverse conditions would be considerably less and you would deteriorate quicker than the Raw Food Eater who never left. With more time you could return home safely, as the *law of adaptation* works both ways. Before leaving the Himalayas, you could slowly introduce larger quantities of food to shield yourself from the effects of going back to polluted air.

For ultimate longevity, it is ideal to very gradually keep moving forward, without ever having to move backward. This principle applies to food intake as well. After one stabilizes out, (because they have been eating a consistent diet for a great amount of time) going backwards by eating more food will have an adverse effect. Our body can adjust to a change in the environment and/or food intake if the process is gradual, not shocking. The downside is that this happens at the expense of our health and longevity. Like a rubber band, the elasticity can snap back, but always with a little less than its original tautness.

4
ELIMINATION
To Perfection and Beyond!

The body is always pushing towards perfection. Ideally, the body would live on air alone, in a "Garden of Eden" environment. Anything less is like swimming in dirty air, or chomping down on a mud sandwich.

An improvement in diet or air quality speeds our progress towards optimal health. As I mention in my book *Raw Spirit,* when we eliminate detrimental foods from our diet COMPLETELY and consistently, this is when our health improves. Health is determined more by what we *do not* eat rather than by what we do eat. *{See Appendix A, "What You Don't Eat".}* Cleansing and detoxification happen in direct proportion with the quality and quantity of foods being eliminated from our diet. Let me write that again. **Cleansing and detoxification happen in direct proportion with the quality and quantity of foods being eliminated.**

When we go to a cleaner environment, we are eliminating poor air from our diet, which has a similar effect as eliminating poor food from our diet. Either way, the results are the same – we are going to detox.

Whether moving forward or backwards, all change to the body is best done gradually. Picture an 85-year-old woman who has a degenerative disease and a lifetime of poor eating behind her. The shock of throwing her into a 100% Raw Food Diet would likely be disastrous due to *autointoxication*.[2] The experienced holistic doctor would know to slowly transition this woman to a better diet and assist her detoxification with frequent Colonic Irrigations.

Extreme caution and care are advisable with improvements to your lifestyle. Dr. Fred Bisci touches on this point in his *Raw Spirit* interview:

Q: *I mention in this book that a Raw Food Eater is more sensitive to polluted air than a cooked food eater. Do you feel your health is suffering because you are a Raw Foodist living in New York's polluted air?*

A: Of course it is not the optimal environment, but the body has about a 20% margin of error and we are able to handle certain things. Not everyone can live in a pristine environment. We have a life to lead. I know a lot of people who retreat to Costa Rica, Ecuador, or some of these other places. They try to live "Garden of Eden" -like lives in the jungle, just living on fruit. Most people I have seen didn't do well at all, and some actually died from trying. I know one person who was paralyzed for a while. They got very sick living mostly on a fruitarian diet. Johnny Lovewisdom thought he was going to succeed at living that way. He moved to Ecuador and died in poor health at about 80 years old. I have seen plenty of people try to do these types of things, thinking they

---

[2] Simply stated, autointoxication literally means "self-poisoning". When we make an extreme improvement to our quantity and/or quality of food, the body's cells can finally dump their tremendous burdens of waste. However, during this massive outpouring, the cells often release more toxins into the bloodstream than can be eliminated at one time. Autotoxemia is the main contributing factor in the case of both mild symptoms and serious disease.

were getting cleaner and cleaner. In my opinion, they didn't really understand the underlying workings of the body...

Later on in the interview he is quoted as saying:

I know some people from the US that went to South America, became Fruitarians. Many lost their teeth and did not do well in the long-run. They couldn't handle the sudden transition from a toxic environment to a very clean location and lifestyle. The release of endogenous [waste inside a cell] material is what harmed them. There was nothing wrong with what they were doing. It was just too much of a change from one extreme to another. They went from a bad environment to a good environment, and a bad diet to a very good diet. Maybe if they would have eaten greens and did Colonics down there it wouldn't have happened to them.

The Base of Our Environment

The planet's air quality has steadily degenerated from centuries of human influence. Over the years, our planet has become polluted. Gradually, we humans have adjusted to this debris; our cells are bathed in it – it is the brown water we swim in. I call this "normal" toxicity saturating our air: *The Base of Our Environment*.

It starts with a puff of exhaust from a diesel truck. As it enters the air, this dark cloud begins to dissipate up and out. At some point we can't even see it anymore. Out of sight, out of mind. We forget about it. But where did it go? Into "The Base of Our Environment". If you add up the collective "puffs" from cigarettes, automobiles, and factories that dissipate, yet remain in our air, you can more fully understand why breathing is like swimming in dirty water. The Base of this dirty environment is the result of gradual degeneration, from centuries of Man's influence here.

The Base of Our Environment does *not* include full-strength contaminants that have not yet dissipated, such as hanging out in the same room with a smoker, being enveloped in a cloud of exhaust, or spending time at an aunt's who lives near a coal factory. At full density, these contaminants are "extras" and not considered part of The Base of Our Environment.

The "excess" toxins periodically added to The Base of Our Environment are eliminated by the body when we combine healthy eating with a few cleansing techniques. *{Cleansing is discussed in Chapter 7.}* As Raw or healthy eaters, we rapidly regenerate, and these "excess" toxins do not affect our long-term health if we are exposed to them infrequently.

The Base of Our Environment varies all across the planet. Although degeneration has occurred globally, certain locations are worse off than others. For instance, The Base of Our Environment in Los Angeles is much more degenerated, brown, and dense compared to The Base of The Environment in the mountains of Mount Shasta, California. *{If you review the diagrams again in Chapter 3 – Optimal Lifestyle, the right side of the diagrams represents The Base of Our Environment.}*

5
HOW DO WE DIGEST FOOD AND AIR?

Is it true that we are what we eat?
Yes. It is also true that we are what we breathe.

"A Breath of Fresh Air"

After all the discussion about air quality, it is valuable to understand a bit about how air is taken in and used by the body.

(1) With every pump of the heart, the liquid going *to* our heart is a combination of CO_2 (carbon dioxide), blood, lymph fluid, and digested nutrients from food. The heart sends this mixture to our lungs. (2) CO_2 is a waste byproduct from our cells, and is poisonous if left in the body, so it quickly gets exchanged for new oxygen from the air we inhale, which includes The Base of Our Environment. (3) Still full of digested nutrients, this newly oxygenated elixir returns to the heart, and then (4) gets distributed to our hungry cells.

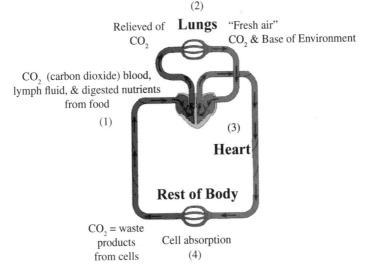

(2)

Relieved of **Lungs** "Fresh air"
CO_2 CO_2 & Base of Environment

CO_2 (carbon dioxide) blood,
lymph fluid, & digested nutrients
from food
(1)

(3)

Heart

Rest of Body

CO_2 = waste
products
from cells

Cell absorption
(4)

Every molecule of oxygen we inhale is drenched with The Base of Our Environment, our "dirty water". This is the "fresh air" that travels through our blood and is absorbed by our cells. There is no escaping the toxic base of our air quality unless you relocate to a cleaner environment.

As we have learned, it is the absence or elimination of toxins that allows the body to go to the next level of health. Since we are continually breathing in this dirty air with each inhale, there is no freedom for our bodies to eliminate it. With every breath, the cells absorb "imperfect" oxygen. In the cell's futile attempt to rid itself of this filth, another round of imperfect oxygen is being delivered with our next inhale. Surrendered, the cell accepts this imperfect oxygen as normal. The cell lowers its standards and submits to this condition as "fresh" air, giving up the fight to improve. The base pollution of our environment is now part of our cells, a part of us. We are a product of our environment.

We Are What We Eat

The same principle applies to eating. For most people, their cells never get a break from the poor quality foods they eat from meal-to-meal. As the cell boldly attempts to eliminate the residue from less-than-optimal meal choices, the next feast of the day is ready to dump its foul garbage into the cell. The cell *becomes* what it cannot eliminate; hence, we are what we eat. Or as one Raw Food Enthusiast puts it, "We are what we don't excrete". If we are to be free of this food toxicity, these harmful foods must be completely omitted from the diet...

eventually and gradually. Only then can our health and vitality soar to the next level.

Excellent Absorption is Essential

There is a scientific explanation for how our cells *absorb food*, which I have mapped out below. You will notice that the process of how our cells absorb the food we eat is similar to how we absorb the air we breathe.

First we eat! Food takes its regular course of digestion from mouth to stomach, and at a certain point passes into the small intestine – over 20 feet of narrow squiggly tubing. From here, broken down food particles are absorbed into microscopic *villi* that line the small intestines. Waiting inside each tiny villi are lacteals (white blood cells) from the lymph system.

(1) Like miniature taxicabs, these lacteals transport food particles through the lymph system to the heart, by way of the thoracic duct and jugular vein superhighway. (2) Other digested food particles in the small intestine are absorbed straight into the blood and by way of the liver, are sent to the heart. These mixtures of digested food particles in the lymph and blood are called *chyle*. The *chyle* from all avenues of the body are gathered and transported first to the heart. (3) Blood laden with waste products from the cells (CO_2) also filters into the heart through various inlets. (4) Everything is sent to the lungs where carbon dioxide waste is exchanged for a fresh supply of oxygen. (5) This newly oxygenated mixture, including nutrients from our food, is finally ready (6) for distribution to the hungry cells.

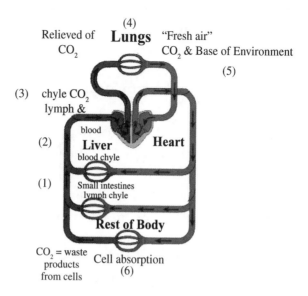

(4) **Lungs**

Relieved of CO_2

"Fresh air" CO_2 & Base of Environment

(5)

(3) chyle CO_2 lymph &

blood

(2) **Liver**   **Heart**

blood chyle

(1) Small intestines
lymph chyle

Rest of Body

CO_2 = waste products from cells   Cell absorption (6)

So you can now see how eating food is similar to breathing polluted air. Both food and air are brought to the cells for absorption by way of the blood. Every inch of us is composed of hundred of thousands of cells. We *are* our cells – we are what we breathe, we are what we eat. Practically speaking, we have considerably more control over what goes in our mouth, versus what goes into our lungs. There is little we can do to improve The Base of Our Environment; however, we can do something about our food choices and the "extra" air pollutants we allow into our space.

6
WHAT ARE WE DETOXING?

What Are We Detoxing?
**Our environment, our food,
our emotions, and our ancestors.**

Incomplete Elimination

Planet Earth has never seen such impurities. The body of Man has never before experienced this densely polluted condition. Every day, every hour, every moment we are bringing foreign toxic chemicals into our bodies. Through the law of adaptation, our bodies are transforming and coping to handle this ever-increasing filth.

Our cells do not eliminate The Base of Our Environment, but they are continually eliminating any additional toxins that suddenly enter our "fresh air", such as clouds of exhaust, vapors from perfumes, and the stench of household cleansing agents. Our cells dispose of this extra waste via the lungs, skin and bowel. It seems to me that if the junk were being *completely* eliminated, we would be walking around with tremendous body odor, gas, and bad breath.

It stands to reason that some toxins are not being eliminated; the body cannot keep up, and the noxious elements are being stored in our cells and tissues. If you are 100% Raw, these un-eliminated poisons are more destructive than they are to the average eater. Our bodies can endure the accumulated toxins for decades with minimal noticeable interference in our quality of life. However, if we want to take this Raw Food Diet to the next level and live beyond the age of 100, something must be done.

The Equation of Longevity

The environment is just one of many factors that Man's body endures. Emotional and spiritual health are also significant elements to include in the equation of longevity. We are under more stress today than ever before, and this is tremendously detrimental to the body. For example, when we experience stressful emotions – anger, fear, jealousy, hatred – our adrenal glands produce adrenalin in excess. The potency of adrenalin becomes poisonous to the human body at this volume.

In addition to emotional and spiritual x-factors, the modern body must also cope with "plastic foods". Prehistoric man's menu never included Snickers® candy bars, processed ingredients, pizza, soda, or Ben & Jerry's Ice Cream®. Even if you are currently 100% Raw, it's likely that you were a "plastic junky" at some point, and still have stored toxins in your cells.

Unloading Generations of Waste

The cells of our great-great-great-great-great-great grandparents, 450 years ago, were *much cleaner* than ours by comparison. It has taken generations to adapt to what we are composed of today, to the abuse we can tolerate. Shockingly, our cells contain inside them the less-than-optimal choices of past generations, which have led to our current condition. At some point in our cleansing, we will be eliminating the poor food choices of our ancestors.

As Raw Foodists, our rigorous cleansing diet releases these age-old (even generational-old) toxins into our bloodstream for elimination, which is a burden most cooked food eaters never need to bear because they do not detox as deeply. Add to this our sensitivity to the environment and the fact that we are more vulnerable to the damage from stress-induced adrenaline, and it is clear why our lifespan suffers.

7
STEP 1: CLEANSING

The Big Question is:
How do we succeed in the long-run as Raw Foodists in the face of all these extra vulnerabilities?
Cleansing.

Our Hope

Thankfully, there are quite a few effective cleansing techniques that can help with our long-term Raw Success, such as an infrared sauna, liver cleanse, foot soaks, salt baths, and the most potent cleansing technique of all – Colonic Irrigations. **The #1 reason why the 100% Raw Food Eater does not succeed in the short and long-run is neglecting to do Colonic Irrigations.**

Our Colon

Our colon is the central waste station of this extraordinary factory we call: a body. Waste products from three meals a day get deposited here. The colon is also the major drop-off spot for any junk eliminated by our organs, toxins from the environment, poisons from stressed out gland secretions, and the millions of cells and tissues which have served their purpose and come here to die. *These cells and tissues are dead proteins of a highly toxic nature if allowed to ferment and putrefy. The colon is our sewage system. Waste accumulates here and not to cleanse it regularly will result in a shorter life than if the cleansing *did* take place. *(*Norman Walker: Colon Health, Pg. 4-5)*

We Must Eliminate

A 100% Raw Food Diet is significantly more cleansing compared to a cooked food diet. Yet, the very best diet is no better than the very worst diet if a thorough elimination of stirred up toxins is not achieved!

The cooked food eater stores toxins in their cells; this is the body's defense against the S.A.D. lifestyle. Conversely, the cells of a 100% Raw Food Eater continually purge a lifetime of stored waste into the bloodstream for elimination through the major channels – skin, lungs, and colon. It is vital that we expel these poisons as soon as possible, so they do not cause fatigue, anxiety, headaches, and damage to our sensitive tissues. Therefore, especially with a Raw Diet, it is highly recommended that we aid our aggressive detox with Colonic Irrigations and other cleansing methods.

The 100% Raw Food Diet Is a Life-Long Fast!

Fasting detoxifies the body because all food is omitted. A Raw Diet detoxifies the body because all food is omitted except Raw Food. In this light, a Raw Diet can be considered a Life-Long Fast.

Most people wouldn't think of undergoing an extended Fast without the simultaneous use of supportive cleansing methods such as Enemas, Colonics, skin brushing, and fresh juices. We realize that to neglect these cleansing aids would make the fasting experience much more exhausting, painful, and even dangerous.

We need to appreciate the similarly aggressive nature of a Fast and a Raw Diet. Many people, even many Raw Pioneers, don't understand this concept and that is one main reason why long-term 100% Raw Food Eaters run into problems. There are numerous instances where Raw Foodists reverted to an 80% - 90% Raw Diet because 100% Raw did not seem to be working for them. Likely, their troubles would have quickly ended if they had done *frequent* colon cleansing.

I Must Be Done Cleansing By Now, Right?

Most people assume that all the old waste from previous years of poor eating leaves their cells within a few short months on a 100% Raw Diet. While it is true that a great amount of toxins are eliminated relatively quickly, the surprising fact is that you are going to detox old waste for the rest of your life! In fact, it is only after many decades being Raw, that you may finally be ready to purge concentrated toxic material passed on to you from your ancestors. We did not get into our current state of toxicity and tolerance overnight, and we will not be magically transported into purity overnight either.

For optimal health, it is imperative to continually keep up with the expulsion of waste matter. Thus, ironic as it may seem, someone who is truly 100% Raw should be getting Colonic Irrigations more often than someone who is not Raw. My recommendation for a 100% Raw Food Eater is a minimum of one irrigation per month. For optimal long-term success, this should continue indefinitely. Those who run into problems on the 100% Raw Diet, often do not know why. Periodic colon cleansing would mean SUCCESS for 95% of these cases.

{The section in the middle of the book, "The Science

Behind It All", shares a deeper explanation about why a 100% Raw Food Diet is a Life-Long Fast. There is a direct correlation between how much one detoxifies and how sensitive they become on a cellular level. Just think of it: I have been detoxing for over seven years, and Dr. Fred Bisci has been detoxing more than 40 years on this Life-Long Fast. For long-term success, it is of the utmost importance that we understand exactly what happens in the body as we detox and why cleansing is so beneficial.}

Why Colonics?

Regardless of whether you have three bowel movements per day (and chances are you do not), there is still waste trapped in your system. Remember, in addition to our solid food waste, there are a host of other toxic substances from 21st Century living, which we were not designed to deal with. Even if 96% of waste leaves our system, the other 4% that is continually left behind will build up day-by-day, week-after-week.

We also must take into account that many of us don't have "perfect" eating habits on the Raw Diet. I witness the strictest Raw Foodists eating between meals. *Having a constant urge to eat between meals suggests an imbalance of the digestive and metabolic functions. If you decide to eat something an hour or two after a meal, the stomach is forced to leave the previously eaten meal half-digested and attend to the newly ingested food. The older food begins to ferment and putrefy, which creates toxemia, gas, and stress throughout the entire digestive tract. Plus, the most recent meal receives inadequate amounts of digestive juices, leaving it only half-digested. *(*Andreas Moritz: The Amazing Liver & Gallbladder Flush, Pg. 77)*

The #1 cause of toxemia is the failure to eliminate toxins from our bodies. Toxins not eliminated are stored primarily in the colon. Before long, the colon reaches saturation point and the poisons spill over into the blood and cellular fluid, causing a host of afflictions.

I have seen numerous people transition to a 100% Raw Diet, and refuse to do Colonics. Due to the deep cleansing effect of Raw Foods, these individuals frequently run into problems with pimples (acne), rashes, hemorrhoids, and other bothers. They are mystified and blame the diet. In reality, they are chock-full of waste that is being forced out through the skin, since the colon is not being sufficiently emptied.

One single Colonic is not the answer. Colonic Irrigation must be done regularly to keep up with the toxic outpouring. The appropriate number of Colonics is unique to the person, their diet, and their condition. For example, if a person was suffering from skin symptoms, I would recommend doing one Colonic every 7-10 days for however long it takes the condition to clear, assuming they are on the 100% Raw Diet and not overdoing sugars. This can take many months. If the individual was not completely Raw, but was willing to eat a healthy transition diet, I would tell them they could succeed at clearing their condition; however, I would warn them that eating harmful foods such as refined sugar and processed starches, even if it were only every once in awhile, would make complete healing impossible.

I am of the strong opinion that the majority of people who are not successful on the 100% Raw Diet could experience a dramatic turn around with Colon Cleansing. There is a documentary about a man who switched from being Vegan to Raw Vegan. The first week he felt like he had won the lottery! After week two, his energy plummeted, he felt depressed, suffered intense cravings for coffee and food that he hadn't consumed in years, and was about to quit. Desperate, he decided to do a Colonic Irrigation. Immediately following this Colonic, he reached a level of well-being he had never before experienced. The Colonic eliminated the accumulating waste, which relieved his cravings and gave him unsurpassed energy. If Colonics had not saved the day, it's very likely he would have abandoned the Raw Diet and returned to a lifelong struggle with dietary bankruptcy.

For the Skeptical Minds

There are those in the Raw and other health communities who are against Colon Cleansing. I have found that many of these folks may claim to be 100% Raw, yet later reveal they eat some cooked food. I believe the percentage of true, 100% Raw Foodists is actually very low. Surprisingly, there is quite a difference in the body of someone who is 95% Raw versus 100% Raw. Someone who is 95% never journeys through the refined sensitivity and profound expulsion of deep-seated waste, and therefore may not appreciate the need for supportive cleansing on a Raw Diet.

Without additional cleansing, toxins are stirred up faster than they are eliminated, resulting in continual cravings and loss of energy. Often, the semi-Raw eater who refuses Colonics is unconsciously forced to compromise their diet, in order to slow down detoxification. It may serve you to keep this in mind the next time someone says they do not need or believe in Colon Cleansing.

It is my deep belief that you are setting yourself up for failure if you are 100% Raw and not doing Colon Hydrotherapy. A Raw Lifestyle is a LIFE-LONG FAST. Without complete elimination, we run the risk of *autointoxication*, a condition in which the cells are giving off more endogenous toxins than are actually being eliminated from the body. Many long-term Raw Foodists do not understand that detox continues for life. Years into a Raw Lifestyle, they may assume that their ill feelings and low energy indicate that a Raw Lifestyle is not for them. In reality they are drowning in their own waste and need a Colonic! This is one of the main reasons why some Raw Pioneers did not live well past the century mark.

I strongly believe that some of those Pioneers were mystified at their health complications. In a last cry for help they returned to a cooked diet, which predictably means the start of a host of afflictions and symptoms, including degenerative disease. After you have *truly* been on a 100% Raw Diet for more than four decades, you become very sensitive and are in danger of shock if wavering from your consistent diet. At this level of evolution, going backwards to a cooked food diet would be like a person on the Standard American Diet inhaling asbestos.

I knew of a man who developed a serious degenerative disease and healed himself by adopting a healthier diet. He was warned that he must eat this way the rest of his life, and that to relapse into his old ways would cause problems. He got married and started eating his wife's food because she would get upset if he didn't eat what she made for him. His degenerative disease came back in full force. Upon getting confirmation from his doctor that his illness had returned, he and his wife both agreed that was the last he'd ever taste of his wife's cooking. Fortunately this man was able to heal once again by adhering to a better diet.

It's Time to Re-Route Doubt

Colonic Irrigations are not natural you say?

Neither is the compromised condition of our planet! Personally, I wouldn't shorten my life because of an outdated principle or philosophy. It has been thrilling for me to witness hundreds of success stories due to Colonic Irrigations. The final pages of this book offer a few real-life testimonials. Before someone writes off the benefits of Colonics, I recommend they try a series themselves first.

So you would rather detox "naturally" and go on a fast, instead of Colon Cleansing?

Fasting can be wonderful; however, it is a crisis-causing situation. If a Raw Food Eater is disturbed because they are clogged with toxins, fasting may just exacerbate the problem. Eliminating all food completely will throw the body and cells into even deeper cleansing. Fasting in this case adds more fuel to the bonfire, whereas Colonic Irrigation would carry the poisons out of circulation and relieve any discomfort.

Can't I use some other healing method and get the same results?

While other cleansing methods are helpful, they are not nearly as effective as Colonic Irrigations. There is a reason for this. If you recall, the colon is the central waste station, the dumping ground for every bit of bodily debris. It follows then that a dirty colon is the "root cause" of most disease and symptoms of ill health. Waste in the colon is like the deeply embedded roots of disease, spreading like a tree throughout the body, affecting the entire system.

Colon flushing is so remarkable that it greatly boosts the potency of other cleansing tools, such as infrared sauna treatment. Getting into a sauna with a dirty colon will indeed skim off some debris. But, if you flush your colon first, removing the thick hodgepodge of waste, and then take a sauna, it affords the body an opportunity for deep cellular cleansing.

Why then do I feel better just by adding more greens to my diet?

It is true that greens are remarkable! They alkalize your body while providing an abundance of precious minerals and nutrients. Adding greens makes the acidic toxins we are eliminating easier to handle. YES, we feel better when we eat more greens; yet that can cause us to assume that greens are the perfect and complete solution to our troubles. However, what is inside the colon must come out. If you are truly 100% Raw and not cleansing your colon frequently, the un-eliminated waste will catch up to you in the long-run.

Why do I have more gas since becoming Raw?

One of the biggest "hidden" complaints among Raw Food Eaters is our ever-present intestinal gas. There are many factors that cause this mysterious gas in the system. The four main factors are: (1) environmental toxins, (2) stress – our emotional health, (3) non-ideal eating habits – overeating, lack of sufficient chewing, overlapping meals, late night snacking, poor food combining, (4) and the ongoing detoxification that will continue until we die because we are on a Life-Long Fast.

If you are living in a pristine environment, stress free, with flawless eating habits, the quantity of gas will be less, yet still present to some degree because of reason #4, our continuous life-long detox. Intestinal gas is one of the costs of striving for perfection in an "imperfect world". Luckily, our rewards make it well worth any annoyances. *{More about the cause of gas can be found in "The Science Behind it All".}*

Do I have to do Colonics?

It is possible to live a long, healthy life on the 100% Raw Diet without Colonic Irrigations. It is unlikely, however, that you will reach extraordinary levels of vitality and longevity past the century mark. I will note that there is no guarantee on long life, even if you have a pristine diet and an impeccable colon. There is more than meets the eye. A life of joy and longevity benefits from discipline and spiritual growth.

With that being said, doing Colonics regularly is absolutely essential for *ultimate* Raw Success. I recommend that a 100% Raw Food Eater do a *minimum* of one Colonic Irrigation per month to keep up with the waste being purged from cells into circulation. Many people do not commit to this many Colonics – they have lower energy, suffer cravings, and become internally clogged. Colonic Irrigation can involve professional Colonics, or at-home devices such as a Colema Board® or a 6-quart Enema bag. Links to these tools can be found in the Resource Guide.

What Else?

What are the other steps necessary to surpass the average life expectancy of mankind? The remainder of *Raw Success* details what I believe are the essential elements to become a vital Centenarian. Raw Food Pioneers are dying between the ages of 80 and 93, or younger! If the Raw Diet is really ideal, we ought to be living decades longer. The only pioneer I know to exceed the 100-year mark is Dr. Norman Walker. After talking with some of those managing the Norwalk family business, it appears they have evidence that Dr. Walker lived 118 years. Regardless of the age to which he truly lived, I feel that he provides an optimal model for long-term health. One of the three core principles for health that Walker encouraged is regular Colonic Irrigations and Enemas. I will be referencing the wisdom of Dr. Walker frequently, to guide us beyond a century of health. It has been a joy to thoroughly study his material so that I could confidently offer you every tool available to ensure your own *Raw Success*.

8
STEP 2: AVOIDING MARGINAL DEFICIENCIES

Can 100% Raw Foodists be deficient in vitamins and minerals?
Absolutely, unless they supplement with a variety of fresh organic vegetable juices.

Vegetable Juicing

It is alarmingly common to meet Raw Foodists with nutritional deficiencies. Tooth decay, hair loss, reduced life span, and other unfortunate consequences have been experienced by many of us on this supposedly ideal lifestyle. Unarguably, the solution in our modern world is: Vegetable Juicing. Habitually juicing a wide variety of vegetables is necessary to catapult us past the century mark with abundant vitality; vegetable juicing is necessary for long-term *Raw Success*.

Recently I met up with a friend who has been Raw for decades. Over the years of our acquaintance he's gotten an earful from me about the importance of vegetable juice. He ate well – he was not in the habit of overeating fruit and ate two or three simple meals throughout the day. Settled in a strict Raw routine, he and even his body resisted juicing. It had been well over a year since we last connected. Something looked different about his appearance, but I could not put my finger on it. He confided that his tooth structure had deteriorated to such an extent that he now had an entire set of false teeth! Sadly, this is not an unusual confession for long-term Raw Foodists.

A 100% Raw Food Diet without juicing vegetables is a deficient diet.

What I am about to share with you is very important and I want it said just right, so I will give a direct passage from *Fresh Vegetable and Fruit Juices* by Dr. Norman Walker:

> *An entirely Raw Food regimen, without the inclusion of a sufficient quantity and variety of fresh-Raw juices is equally deficient. The reason for this deficiency lies in the fact that a surprisingly large percentage of the atoms making up the nourishment in the Raw Foods is utilized as fuel for energy by the digestive organs in their processes of digesting and assimilating the food, which usually requires as long as 3, 4, or 5 hours after every meal. Such atoms, while furnishing some nourishment to the body, are mostly used up as fuel, leaving only the smaller percentage available for the regeneration of the cells and tissues.*
>
> *However, when we drink Raw vegetable juices, the situation is entirely different, as these are digested and assimilated within 10 to 15 minutes after we drink them and they are used almost entirely in the nourishment and regeneration of the cells and tissues, glands and organs of the body. In this case the result is obvious, as the entire process of digestion and assimilation is completed with a maximum degree of speed and efficiency, and with a minimum of effort on the part of the digestive system.*
>
> (Norman Walker: Fresh Vegetable and Fruit Juices, Pg. 9)

Juicing a *wide variety* of vegetables is the optimal

way to supply the vitamins and minerals we need. Our bodies love veggie juice! The liquid flows straight into our small intestines, and is easily absorbed. Juicing is the best, most natural way to get vitamins and minerals in their most absorbable form ~ liquid, liquid, LIQUID! Try for a minimum of two 16oz vegetable juices every day.

Juicing vs. Blending?

Blending our fruits and vegetables can be a wonderful way to prepare Raw Food. Blended food digests easier as it is already broken down. Additionally, blending bursts the cell walls of fruits and vegetables, making more nutrients available to the body than our teeth could release because of insufficient chewing. However, blending is *NOT* a replacement for juicing. Juiced foods are exponentially easier to assimilate because all fiber and solids are removed. Juice is simply and perfectly – liquid. Unlike a blended salad, with juicing, every bit of nourishment can be used to regenerate rather than digest.

Be diligent to chew blended foods. It can be tempting to quickly swallow blended meals because there is nothing solid to break down with our teeth. However, if there is any amount of fiber present in your meal, chewing is necessary to prepare the stomach for digestion. Neglecting this step can cause imperfect or partial absorption, not to mention gas and bloating. If you are going to blend, I recommend "chewing" each mouthful until it is thoroughly salivated and trickles down the esophagus on its own without you consciously swallowing.

Norman Walker is in complete agreement with this concept. He writes:

A blender is not practical for the extraction of juices. Its action merely cuts up the vegetables as fine as desired, but the pulp is still present in its entirety. Furthermore, to drink juices from which the pulp has not been extracted taxes the digestive organs more than eating and properly masticating the Raw vegetables and fruits themselves, as proper insalivation and thorough mastication is essential to the complete digestion of vegetables when the cellulose fiber is present. This is not usually done if the fibers still remain a part of the mush or liquefied vegetables; whereas, the juices from which the fiber has been removed furnish, without interference, every particle of the nourishment contained in the vegetable for immediate and quick assimilation by the body.

(Norman Walker: Fresh Vegetable and Fruit Juices, Pgs. 14 &16)

Which Juicers are Best?

The best juicer is one that you are going to consistently use. A juicer choice takes into account your finances, the time you are willing to devote to juicing/cleaning, and your desire for longevity. I personally use the Norwalk Juicer for its superb nutrient quality – every possible atom of nutrition is squeezed into my glass. Also, because of its advanced juice extraction methods, fresh Norwalk juices can be refrigerated and kept for up to three days, unlike some other extraction methods which produce juice that spoils if not consumed within 15 minutes.

The Norwalk Juicer, created by Norman Walker himself, is an exceptional machine designed for the most complete

The Science
Behind It All

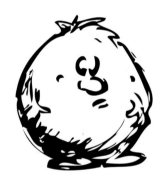

The Blood Gas Theory

ACKNOWLEDGMENT

What I am about to share was inspired by my mentor, Dr. Fred Bisci. Fred started planting seeds in my head years ago. The harvest of their fruit, I share with you. Take what you can use and leave the rest for another day.

THE GAS MYSTERY UNVEILED

Many people, especially Raw Foodists, are often befuddled about what gas is and why it can sometimes seem never ending. Flatulence or raucous belching is not necessarily part of our "Garden of Eden" fairytale. The answer to this mysterious gas lies within our cells. The well-kept secret has eluded so many because cells are small and mysterious, not to mention completely hidden within and beneath our wonderful skin.

What is actually happening inside us on a cellular level?
Our cells are full of gas.

Gas is a result of fermentation. Normal digestion always results in a certain amount of fermentation; it is a natural and inevitable byproduct of digestion. With that being said however, we do have control over the amount of gas produced. The quality, quantity, and combinations of foods we eat determine the amount of fermentative gas released into our system. When this gas is released, our cells absorb it into their structure and it gets "locked in", through the process of something called: *diffusion.*

Gas diffusion – Cell membranes are the boundaries between the internal and external environments of a cell. Diffusion across this cellular membrane is the movement of gas molecules from a region of higher concentration to a region of lower concentration.

Study the diagrams on the following pages for a clearer concept of diffusion.

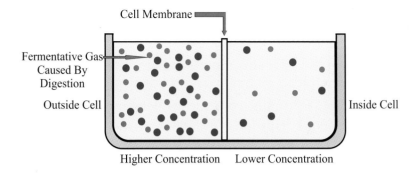

Cell Membrane

Fermentative Gas
Caused By
Digestion

Outside Cell

Inside Cell

Higher Concentration   Lower Concentration

Movement of gas molecules from a region of higher concentration
(outside the cell) to a region of lower concentration (inside the cell)

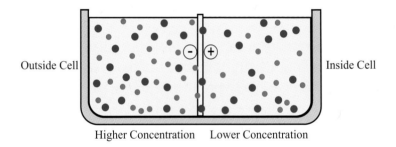

Outside Cell

Inside Cell

Higher Concentration   Lower Concentration

Once gas pressure inside and outside of the cell reaches equilibrium, gas
molecules stop traveling in or out. At equilibrium, the fermentative gas
from eating food gets "locked in" to the cell's structure.

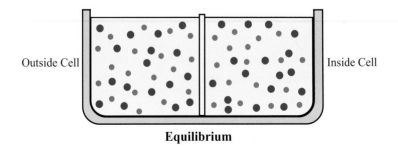

Outside Cell

Inside Cell

Equilibrium

The cells must enlarge to accommodate excessive amounts of incoming gas pressure. The poorer our eating habits, the more fermentative gases are released in our system, and the more abnormally enlarged our cells become.

The cells are continually working to rid themselves of this gaseous waste. However, with non-stop cooked and junky foods, our inflated cells are constantly subjected to elevated levels of fermentative gas, which keep the cells distended.

When someone improves his or her diet, the fermentation decreases considerably.

"Because they are alive and vital,
raw foods do not ferment as readily as cooked foods."
(Dr. St. Louis Estes, Raw Food and Health, Pg. 114)

With a diet of Raw Food, there is literally less (gas) pressure on the cell and, through the same process of gas diffusion, the cell is finally free to contract and release any accumulated toxins and gaseous waste.

You just learned what is actually happening inside the body when someone says they are **detoxing!!!**

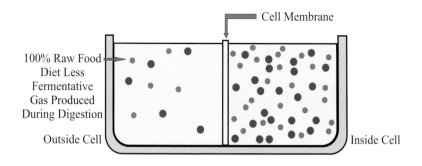

Cell Membrane

100% Raw Food Diet Less Fermentative Gas Produced During Digestion

Outside Cell

Inside Cell

Detoxification

Movement of gas molecules from a region of higher concentration (inside the cell) to a region of lower concentration (outside the cell)

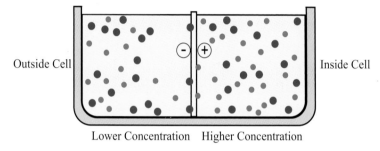

Outside Cell

Inside Cell

Lower Concentration   Higher Concentration

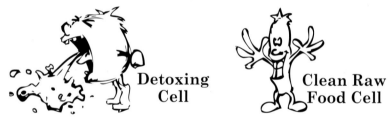

Detoxing Cell

Clean Raw Food Cell

{As you study and gain a deep understanding of this process, you will soon understand the power behind Colon Hydrotherapy.}

Our level of cellular gas has a massive effect on our health and well-being. Perhaps you are saying to yourself, *"It's just a tiny cell, what is the big deal if it's a little gasey?"* The body is made up of an incredible, mind-boggling number of cells; every bit of us consists of cells – our blood, organs, skin, nails, all matter in the body. Yes cells are small, but en masse, a little bit of gaseous waste pouring from thousands of trillions of troopers simultaneously is a big deal.

The process of detoxification (cells contracting to rid themselves of stored gaseous waste) continues for life, especially if one is consistent with an improved diet. Over time, the cells contract more and more, continuing to give off greater quantities of gaseous waste.

Here is a visual comparison:
- Cells on a SAD diet are the size of a large yoga ball

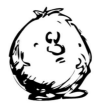

- Cells on a vegetarian diet for 5 years are the size of a basketball

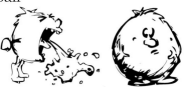

- Cells on a vegan diet for 5 years contract to the size of a soccer ball

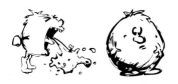

- Cells on a 100% Raw Vegan Diet for 1 year (consistently) shrink to baseball size

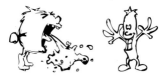

- Cells on a 100% Raw Vegan Diet for 10 years detox to the size of a ping-pong ball

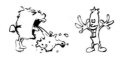

- Cells on a 100% Raw Vegan Diet for 40 years reduce to the size of a marble

- Cells on a 100% liquid diet for 40 years are the size of a microscopic dot or pin prick

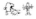

Yo-Yo Dangers

This next section explains why it is so harmful to yo-yo between eating styles or try to move out of the "rabbit hole" too quickly. *{The "rabbit hole" concept is explained in Chapter 13}*

Our body adjusts to what we do consistently, over time. It took years for our cells to gradually expand so that they could accommodate the tremendous amount of fermentative gas pressures from the foods we were eating. Because of the adaptation abilities of our body, we could scarf down more dangerous selections and quantities of food in our twenties than we could as young children.

Digesting cooked meat or processed starches generates considerably more fermentation than digesting Raw Food. **This fermentative gas can damage cells if they are not large enough and don't have the open space to withstand the pressure.**

It is the size of your cells that determines the amount of shock the body experiences. Depending on the cleanliness of your cells, a cheeseburger or slice of cooked apple pie could either mean a nice full belly, an upset tummy and headache, or a one-way trip to the hospital.

To really illustrate the effects, let me break it down again.

The fermentation from a cooked starch/meat meal would result in:

- No effect on the SAD dieter. There is plenty of space in the cell for gas pressure. Bring it on!

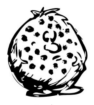

- A bit of fatigue perhaps for the "basketball" vegetarian, still far from any danger zone.

- Headache or nausea for the soccer ball vegan; the gases would fit very snugly and the cell may have to expand a bit to make room.

- Varying levels of illness for the baseball 1-yr Raw Vegan and the ping pong 10-yr Raw Vegan, as the gas pressure shocks and pushes past the cells' capacity.

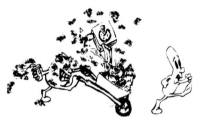

- Massive disaster for the marble 40-yr Raw Vegan and pin-prick Liquidarian. There is no feasible room inside the cell to accommodate the onslaught of gases and the result is detrimental shock.

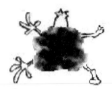

Becoming "too sensitive" can become an issue in the long-run. That is the main reason why I don't encourage people to go beyond the *Optimal Raw Diet* outlined in Chapters 9 & 10. The smaller our cells, the more sensitive we are to damaging environmental toxins and inconsistencies in diet. When someone goes beyond a Liquidarian diet and is practically living on air alone, it's almost impossible to fathom how sensitive and refined that being becomes. In the long-run, their cells would become so extremely small that the gas pressure caused by adverse environmental conditions could have a detrimental effect on their health.

Feeling the Pressure

Do not think that the "basketball-sized" cells of a typical American dieter are immune to consequences. They may be able to endure adverse conditions with little noticeable reaction, but as evidenced by all the illness in today's world, they are clearly suffering from gradual autointoxication. Poor diet combined with less-than-ideal eating habits – junky foods, harmful substances, eating all day without breaks, meals late at night – make degenerative disease inevitable in the long-run.

Massive quantities of fermentation plague the system from poor food and eating habits. Even with three bowel movements a day, and release from belching and flatulence, gas is being packed away. The gas pressure builds in the bloodstream to the point where the cells clog, and are unable to release their carbonic acid gaseous waste due to the principle of gas diffusion explained above. The body is storing more gas than it's releasing. Think of the individuals walking around with enlarged abdomens, like balloons ready to pop. This type of person may be moving their bowels three times a day, yet they are chronically constipated on a cellular level. **Detoxification - getting rid of gaseous cellular waste - is crucial for a healthy disease-free life.**

Lifesaving Detox

You've already learned that the digestive system breaks down food so that nutrients can enter the bloodstream. The bloodstream carries these nutrients to the trillions of hungry cells throughout our body. Looking a bit closer, science has shown that through the process of [1]cellular respiration, the cells convert this fuel (sugar) to useable energy (ATP).[2]

In a healthy body, this is generally done in the presence of oxygen. When oxygen is not available, the cells must use a back-up system that involves anaerobic (absence of oxygen) pathways for converting sugar into energy. This back up system is *fermentation*. Knowing what we know about the damaging effects of fermentation, you can probably see the disastrous direction this is heading.

Why are we forced to use a back-up system; why wouldn't oxygen be available to convert sugar to energy?

Detoxification - getting rid of gaseous cellular waste - is crucial for a healthy, disease-free life. If a person is chronically constipated on a cellular level, the cells can't release their gaseous waste (Remember diffusion – if the pressure on the outside of the cell is the same or greater than the pressure on the inside of the cell, all movement STOPS flowing towards the area of greater pressure). If a cell cannot release this toxic gas, it will expand beyond its natural point of suppleness.

---

[1] Cellular Respiration: This is how cells obtain energy from nutritious molecules. During cellular respiration, energy (ATP) is released and carbon dioxide is produced and absorbed by the blood, to be transported to the lungs.

2 ATP stands for Adenosine Triphosphate.

Whether there is an *absolute* maximum capacity to which the cell can expand from excess gas is a mystery. However, when there is constant excess gas pressure in the bloodstream *and* inside the cell, that cell can get cut off from oxygen. The oxygen can't make its way to the cell through the elevated levels of gas pressure.

So now the cells have to use anaerobic (absence of oxygen) pathways to convert fuel into energy (ATP). Instead of using oxygen to create energy, the anaerobic process generates alcohol fermentation and lactic acid fermentation to produce energy. If this process continues for extended periods of time, it is destructive to tissue and can result in inflammation, which later develops into the host of degenerative diseases all too common in today's world.

The Cause of Cancer – Explained

In 1931 Otto Warburg was awarded the Nobel Prize in Physiology. Otto Warburg is known for discovering the cause of cancer. He stated, *"The prime cause of cancer is the replacement of the respiration of oxygen (oxidation of sugar) in normal body cells by fermentation of sugar."* He is saying that the prime cause of cancer is when the body is forced to use anaerobic pathways to convert fuel (sugar/glucose) to energy. Ding! Ding!

An article entitled "The Scientific Basis Behind Alternative Cancer Treatments", by Tanya Harter Pierce, MA, MFCC states:

Otto Warburg demonstrated that all cancer cells share the important trait of being primarily anaero-

bic. Whereas all healthy cells in our bodies require an oxygen-rich environment. Warburg was able to show that cancer cells actually thrive in an oxygen-depleted environment. He further proved that, rather than using oxygen, cancer cells use glucose fermentation for their energy needs.

The reason that healthy cells sometimes change from aerobic respiration to anaerobic respiration – and then may turn into cancer cells – is not entirely understood.

The theory I propose above explains what "is not entirely understood". The article goes on to theorize:

However, it is known that under stress, the tissues of the body have a tendency to become more acidic then they would otherwise be. It is also known that oxygen is less able to be assimilated by the body as the cellular environment becomes more acidic. Therefore as the body is stressed by any number of means, such as poor nutrition, toxins, physical stress, or dehydration, the cells of the body may adopt anaerobic respiration as a survival mechanism.

In actuality, poor nutrition, toxins and physical stress create the gas pressure which puts the tissue of the body under stress causing a more acidic condition. At this point, the oxygen is less able to be assimilated by the body.

Once in the more primitive anaerobic state, these cells no longer function efficiently and many of the natural mechanisms that control cell division break down, sometimes resulting in cancer. Based on these scientific facts, some of the most effective alternative cancer therapies exploit the cancer cell's dependency on anaerobic functioning. High pH Therapy and some Nutritional/Dietary Therapies seek to reduce the acidity of the cancer cell and surrounding environment to remove the conditions in which the cancer thrives.

The goal is not to reduce the acidity of the body. It is to relieve the body of this gas pressure which will result in a less acidic condition. The two most effective ways to accomplish this task are adhering to a healthier diet, while undertaking Colon Hydrotherapy. When you eat a healthier diet, less fermentative gas is produced in your bloodstream during digestion. This lowers the gas pressure on the outside of the cells. Through the process of diffusion, these gases exit the cells and rapidly discharge into the bloodstream. Colon Hydrotherapy removes this heavy outpour of gaseous waste from the bloodstream, which keeps the gas pressure levels in the bloodstream down, allowing even more cellular detoxification. The release of this backed-up gas pressure will allow oxygen to once again exist within the cells' environment. With more oxygen, the body is not forced to resort to anaerobic, acid-producing fermentation for energy production.

[3]Two other powerful components to aid in cellular detoxification are vegetable juicing and enzyme therapy.

Colon Hydrotherapy

I think you would agree that there are many big-bellied people who have spent decades eating a Standard American Diet. Many of these individuals seek out the 100% Raw Food Diet. At first, their results are fantastic. They lose 50 pounds and have incredible energy. As time goes by and the detox goes deeper, however, these same individuals lose energy, don't feel well, get a runny nose, and their face starts to look older. They are bathing in their own waste, even if their bowels are emptying three times a day. This is the type of person who is chronically constipated on a cellular level, due to this overwhelming gas pressure. **They need Colon Hydrotherapy to keep up with all that is being excreted by the cells.** If not willing to do Colon Hydrotherapy, I would highly suggest they get off the CLEANSING 100% Raw Food Diet and instead adopt a healthy transition diet.

It is true that Colonics remove the build up of solid waste from our colon. What most people are not aware of, however, is that solid waste removal is not the main objective! Many colon machines have a viewing window where you can look at what is coming out of your colon during the session. In addition to solid waste, you can also see many tiny bubbles leaving the body. The bubbles are carbonic acid gaseous waste! That is what we are most interested in releasing.

---

3 Juicing will help to alkalinize the acidic toxins entering into the bloodstream, making the experience much more pleasant while also exceedingly nourishing for you (See Chapter 8).   Enzymes will help remove toxins and disease, while repairing damage done to the body (See Chapter 11).

There have been many examples of people's rings falling off their fingers during a Colonic. Why does this happen? That solid matter, our finger, is like a jigsaw puzzle, comprised of thousands of miniature puzzle-piece cells. Over the years, our cells have expanded and become bigger to accommodate a certain amount of carbonic acid gaseous waste. **When these clogged people did a Colonic, they "unclogged the sink" and that gaseous waste was free to leave their cells through the process of diffusion.** This outpouring of carbonic acid gas allowed the cells to contract and become smaller, which literally shrunk their fingers, causing rings to fall off. They deflated! Can't you sometimes see when people are kind of inflated in their face, fingers, or ankles and could benefit enormously from getting this done?

Colon Hydrotherapy is an invaluable tool for all people, regardless of their lifestyle and eating habits, particularly because it allows for our cells to return to the "lean" state that is in alignment with the way our bodies were designed to thrive.

Gas and Ailments

Dr. St. Louis Estes, author of *Raw Food and Health*, is the only other author I know of who seemed to have an understanding of these blood gas concepts. His book is listed in the Resource Guide. I highly recommend reading the chapter entitled "Gases". He writes:

Gas in the stomach and in the bowels is a chronic disorder characteristic of the reaction of cooked foods.

The organs of the body are thwarted in their functions, displaced, prolapsed and diseased through accumulations of gas, which are generated by putrefying foods.

If you read in-between the lines, you will come to understand that all the organs of the body are overwhelmed and compromised by gas pressure *inside and outside* the cells. He is also saying it is a result of eating cooked food, which causes more putrefying fermentative gas in the system than Raw Food.

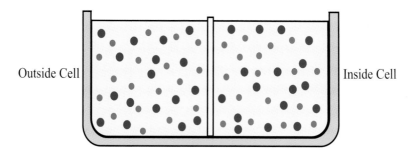

Outside Cell   Inside Cell

Gas is EVERYWHERE, weakening our body with constant stress.

He goes on to write:

People eat a hearty meal and perhaps immediately, or several hours afterward, are annoyed with eructations of gas. They accept this condition as a matter of course and go on from day to day, not realizing that the constant accumulations of gas are pursuing their course back and forth through the body, are greatly increased with every meal, crowd the organs, distend and dislodge them from their normal positions and cause innumerable diseases and disorders and much misery.

The body is consumed with gas pressure inside and outside the cells, organs, and all throughout the body. The gases are actually traveling throughout our blood and are causing the majority of diseases today! Read below:

These gases, though they are indifferently regarded, have a very definite power in undermining the health, depleting the nervous system to such an extent that weakness, loss of memory, vertigo, eye troubles, depression, hysteria and even paralysis, where the pressure is so intense that a large blood vessel gives way.

Even Heart Attacks! :

Palpitation of the heart is very often caused by intestinal gases. I have seen cases suffering from gas pains to such an extent they were forced to go to a hospital for treatment. Every morsel of food or drink which they took into their body was seemingly converted into gas, and the misery which they suffered was intense. Severe contraction of the muscles around the heart and sharp, stubborn pains through the heart areas, which actually shut off the breath for a few seconds, frightened these patients into believing that death was imminent. The natural result of this condition, if neglected, would be a diseased condition of the heart, for the pressure of the gas on the nerves causes surcharging and congestion of the blood vessels and a persistent irritation to the regions afflicted. The great strain on the heart under these circumstances lowers its vitality and changes the heartbeat, making it slower and irregular, or quickened with frequent rapid flutterings and racing throb. Fainting fits are not uncommon to these conditions, for the sudden congestions due to gas around the heart draws the blood from the brain.

And Hair Loss:

Continuous recurrence of this reaction to gas deprives the scalp of its nourishment, and the hair dies and falls out.
(Raw Food and Health, by Dr. St. Louis Estes, Pgs. 112-113)

Extra care is advisable here for those who adhere to the cleansing, 100% Raw Food Diet *(See the section, "The 100% Raw Food Diet Is a Life-Long Fast!" in Chapter 7).* As the years go on, the cells will continually outpour their gaseous waste into the bloodstream. Repeatedly, people who adhere to a 100% Raw Lifestyle confide in me. Many of these people express to me that their hair is falling out. This is a particularly common trait amongst heavy fruit eaters, who develop excess gas from all the fermentation in their system.

Feeling Gasey?

You can now see why gas is continually present in the body of a 100% Raw Food Eater. Aside from the environmental toxins, stress, and poor eating habits, we will forever have a certain amount of gas from the ongoing detoxification (life-long fast), which will continue until we die.

Thankfully, there are ways to minimize the amount of gas in our cells. Cleansing, exercising, keeping stress-free, avoiding environmental toxins, and the most important contributing factor in our control: improving our eating habits. Food combining is one improvement we can make. Even more effective however is not eating late at night, overeating, overlapping meals, or eating all day long. Furthermore, lack of chewing is probably the leading cause of gas in the body of a Raw Foodist.

Chewing Our Food

For those of you just starting a 100% Raw Lifestyle, the practice of Fletcherizing (chewing to a liquid or creamy consistency) each bite of food could take years to perfect and that is absolutely OK. It is a goal to work towards. Expect some possible challenges. One is forced to minimize food intake when Fletcherizing. Not only will you be the last one sitting at the table with a smaller meal, but it will generally take you five times longer than it did before to finish a meal. Your loved ones will have finished eating, washed their dishes and accomplished ten other things, in the time it takes you just to eat.

Dr. St. Louis Estes writes:

ALL FOODS will cause gas unless they are thoroughly masticated. If the food is swallowed in chunks, the stomach is absolutely incapable of dissolving that food so that more than a meager percentage of it can be absorbed. The result is that the undigested chunks of food lie inert and heavy, and fermentation shortly begins, followed thereafter by flatulence and discomfort and frequently intense pain.

The GREATEST CARE should be exercised by those living or contemplating living on a diet of RAW FOODS. Because of their highly nutritious properties and the fact that they are eaten in their natural state, with none of the minerals lost, the raw foods have enormous power and are capable of causing great digestive disturbance unless they are thoroughly ground to a creamy consistency with the teeth.

(Raw Food and Health, by Dr. St. Louis Estes, Pgs. 114-115)

For 95% of the Raw Foodists reading this book, Fletcherizing will be an improvement in diet. Eating your exact same meals, Fletcherized, will produce less fermentative gas. With less gas pressure in the body, the cells now have a chance to excrete more of their stored gaseous waste, through the process of diffusion.

Initially, this move forward may result in excessive gas and feelings of detox, until your body stabilizes at its new level of health and vitality.

Science and Spiritual Energy

When you consistently eat a 100% Raw Diet, you are automatically thrown into the more "subtle" realms of life. The body vibrates with increased spiritual energy. This heightened state seems to be in direct proportion to the size of our cells! The smaller our cells, the more receptive we become. Cell "shrinkage" is determined by our cleanliness on a cellular level as well as the cleanliness of our bloodstream.

There are two areas of cleanliness to consider and both are needed for ultimate spiritual receptivity:

1. Cellular Cleanliness
2. Bloodstream Cleanliness

Cellular Cleanliness

The 100% Raw Diet is a Life-Long Fast. As the years go by, our cells continually detox, shrinking the cells more and more. The longer one is Raw, the more purified the cells become and the more the body vibrates with increased spiritual energy.

Bloodstream Cleanliness

The cells of anyone in detox are continually purging and dumping gas into the bloodstream. This cellular dumping affects the second factor: bloodstream cleanliness. If our cellular garbage is not continually being eliminated from the bloodstream (via cleansing such as Colon Hydrotherapy), our cells will not be able to dump as much. If the trashcan is full, the garbage starts to collect in the house. If we continue to neglect our bloodstream, at some point the cells will be forced to reabsorb their discarded waste, plus whatever new obstructions have accumulated in the body. The cells grow larger, to house the increased toxicity, and this cellular expansion compromises spiritual receptivity.

Additionally, toxic *obstructions* that are not eliminated cause a loss of vitality and the body's vibrational spiritual energy lessens. When the bloodstream is free of obstruction, our minds are sharper, the body's bloodstream is purified, and we are brought closer to those cosmic forces.

Obstructions

Arnold Ehret writes in detail about these Obstructions while describing his renowned Formula of Life:

$$\text{"V"} = \text{"P"} - \text{"O"}$$

Vitality = Power – Obstruction

"O" means OBSTRUCTION, encumbrance, foreign matters, toxemias, mucus; in short, all internal impurities which obstruct the circulation, the function of internal organs especially, and the human engine in its entire functioning system.

(Mucusless Diet Healing System, by Arnold Ehret, Pg. 53)

Obstruction is a major deciding factor in both *cellular cleanliness* and bloodstream cleanliness. In terms of cellular cleanliness, the longer you have been on a 100% Raw Vegan Diet, the more your cells detox, shrink and eliminate obstructions within their structure. The majority of cellular obstruction is trapped gaseous waste.

In the case of *bloodstream cleanliness,* during a cell's purification process, it dumps any waste into the bloodstream. Thus, the blood must be regularly cleared of obstructions, such as little dumpings from our trillions of cells. There are many effective cleansing habits to purify the blood – Colon Hydrotherapy, skin brushing, exercising, infrared sauna, etc.

The cleanliness of our bloodstream is also affected by:
◊   Quantity of foods – meal size, meal frequency, raw or dense cooked, etc.
◊   Eating habits – Fletcherizing, overlapping, overeating, etc.
◊   Stress & Environment

All these points mentioned above can produce excessive gas if they are out of balance. The less we eat and the more optimal our lifestyle, the less fermentative gas we have. Less fermentative gas means reduced obstructions in our bloodstream. Conversely, a clogged bloodstream slows down cellular detox because the tremendous gas pressure against the cells is too great. As explained above by the *gas diffusion* principle, the lower the gas pressure outside a cell, the more the cell can purge its waste, enabling it to then purify and shrink. Ultimately, smaller cells result in heightened divine connectivity.

Taking Out The Trash
Cleansing the colon is the #1 way to ensure bloodstream cleanliness and cellular cleanliness. Remember that the colon is the central waste station of the body, the trashcan for all our junk. Colon Hydrotherapy is like taking out the trash. Cleansing the colon empties any gas and waste that may be present and creates a now-empty five-foot long receptacle for the toxins of the body to pour into.
Removing these obstructions from the body allows

for increased purification of the bloodstream and thus, heightened spiritual receptivity. Additionally, due to the process of gas *diffusion*, Colon Hydrotherapy lessens the gas pressure and enables our cells to continually purify – further increasing our spiritual receptivity.

Here is my Formula for Life:
Less Obstruction = Higher Spiritual Receptivity
How does Heaven on Earth sound?

Final Words

This planet is full of good people with good hearts…this book is an attempt to end needless feelings of suffering, for those attempting to make it in this world of confusing "do"s and "don't"s. *Well, here is another Don't:* **Do not take my word for any of this! Improve your own diet and experience the results for yourself.**

juice extraction possible. The Norwalk Juicer is the only triturating juicer that splits open every cell of every fiber, to release the precious nutritional elements. The juice is then pressed through a fine cloth bag, which prohibits any fiber from entering the juice.

A Greenstar twin-gear Juicer® is the next best, and is a very acceptable alternative to the Norwalk Juicer. The Resource Guide in the back of this book offers support to acquire what will serve you best.

Strain Your Juice

Juicing is so effective because it is pure liquid. Assimilating vegetable juice puts absolutely no stress on the body and requires minimal effort to digest. Without fiber or solids, we can achieve maximum absorption of nutrients. Removing all fiber from the juice is essential and very easy. You can simply strain your juice through a nut milk bag or fine-mesh strainer.

Also good to note is that when there are contaminants present in our fruits and vegetables, these toxins get stored in the fiber. Because the Norwalk Juicer removes all the fiber, you do not need to worry about toxins in your vegetable juice. Whenever I am using any other type of juicer, I use a nut milk bag to strain the excess pulp out of the juice. See the Resource Guide for details on ordering nut milk bags.

Many, many, many Veggies

Variety is key to ensure you receive the full spectrum of essential vitamins and minerals. Every vegetable has a different composition of nutrients. Below is a selection of juices that best support long-term Raw Success.

Juice Combinations

As I mentioned previously, to assist our long-term Raw Success, I would be referencing the wisdom of a Raw Pioneer who lived to be 118 years old. His name is Dr. Norman Walker. He spent his life scientifically researching the body and its response to foods and juices. Dr. Walker was never shy about saying that an entirely Raw Food regimen, without the inclusion of a sufficient quantity and variety of fresh Raw juices, is as equally deficient as a cooked food diet. There are several beneficial recipe combinations in his book, "Fresh Vegetable and Fruit Juices." I recommend purchasing this book for further education and support.

A brief note about Dr. Walker:

Reading Dr. Norman Walker's book, *Become Younger*, was the catalyst that convinced me overnight to abandon my SAD diet for Raw Living. Dr. Walker was deathly ill at a youthful age and discovered the power of Raw juicing at a farmhouse in France where he grated carrots and squeezed them through a fine cloth. Feeling the rejuvenating effects, he continued this "re-inventing the wheel" tedious juice extraction until completely cured of all prior illness. His life's mission was then to offer the world the incredible healing power of juicing and live foods. After reading his books, Dr. Walker strikes me as a gentle man, fiery with passion for life and truth. His heart sought to befriend us all and share what he learned, so that we might enjoy our time here even more. Norman Walker fought for Life - yours and mine. To ensure your *Raw Success*, the following chapters contain much wisdom from this remarkable ally.

Green Juices!

- High in chlorophyll
- Provide longer life, beautiful skin, and life force

Carrot Juice – Many people shy away from carrot juice because they are concerned about the sugar content. Carrots have less sugar compared to most fruits such as apples. I personally use carrots in 95% of my green juice combinations to help make them taste better. I would rather use carrots than apples because the nutrient content is exceedingly more beneficial to the body. A few of the carrot juice benefits are listed below.

- Not only is its nutritional value unsurpassed, but also it makes mixtures taste amazing
- Helps normalize the entire system
- Very high in Vitamin A, more than any other vegetable
- Also includes Vitamins B, C, D, E, G, and K
- Helps promote the appetite and assists digestion
- Improvement and preservation of the bone structure of teeth
- A personal favorite of Dr. Walker's; his book *Fresh Vegetable and Fruit Juices* has an entire section dedicated to the benefits of carrot juice

Carrot-Spinach – Intuitively, I feel that spinach is one of the best dark leafy greens we can juice. I drink spinach in my vegetable juices almost every day.

- Extremely beneficial for optimal functioning of the digestive system

- Provides Man with the organic nutrients needed for cleansing, rebuilding, and regeneration of the intestinal tract
- "I'm strong to the finish, 'cause I juice me spinach!"

Carrot-Spinach-Celery-Parsley
- Rich in potassium.
- Reduces excessive acidity in the stomach
- *"There is probably no food more complete and perfect for the human organism. The organic minerals and salts in this combination embrace practically the entire range of those required by the body." (*Norman Walker: *Fresh Vegetable and Fruit Juices*, Pg 49)

Celery
- High in essential organic sodium
- Rich in magnesium and iron
- Ideal nourishment for the blood cells

Carrot-Beet-Cucumber
- Effective for cleansing and healing the gall bladder, liver, kidneys, prostate and other sex glands.

Carrot-Dandelion-Turnip Greens
- High in calcium and magnesium
- Turnip greens have more calcium than any other vegetable. With the high magnesium content (needed to assimilate calcium) in dan-

delion and the other properties of carrot, this juice is ideal for those dealing with a calcium deficiency; it is the best calcium supplement one can take!
- Strengthens teeth and fortifies bone structure of the entire body
- The taste can be strong. One option is to drink the greens and follow with carrot juice

In addition to the above combinations, I juice a variety of seasonal veggies to ensure the fullest spectrum of nutrients possible. Dark leafy greens are incredibly beneficial. When someone drinks green juices I can see that smooth glowing beauty in their skin. The *greatest beauty secret on Earth* is to drink green vegetable juices and regularly cleanse the colon.

Vegetable juicing is the #1 action you can take to avoid deficiencies. In my very loud opinion, based on experience, study, and mass testimonials, **To Not Juice Is A Huge Mistake.**

It is understandable to assume that a healthy diet will give us all the nutrients we need. *Deficiency* is not a common word uttered from the lips of a Raw Foodist. Yet, because of insufficient chewing, depleted soil, limited access to fresh organic foods, our polluted environment and heightened levels of stress, the issue of deficiency is real – for us all. In the next chapter I will continue to problem-solve this roadblock and offer certain foods and supplement suggestions that are important additions to Juicing.

Organic?

Eating mainly organic produce is key for long-term success on the 100% Raw Food Diet. It is a good goal to aim for, no matter which diet you follow. There are many reasons to choose organic; here are a few at the top of my list:

1.   Organic produce is not covered in a thick glob of poisonous chemicals. The average conventionally-grown apple has 20-30 artificial poisons on its skin, even after rinsing.

2.   Fresh organic produce contains on average 50% more vitamins, minerals, enzymes and other micro-nutrients than intensively farmed produce. We want to get as many vital nutrients as possible to avoid deficiencies in the long-run.

3.   Conventional growing methods can seriously damage farm workers' health. There are much higher instances of cancer, respiratory problems and other major diseases amongst farm workers from non-organic farms.

4.   The Deliciousness Factor: organic produce simply tastes better. Conscientious farmers give fruit and vegetables more time on the branch, leaving our produce full of juice and flavor.

9
STEP 3: OPTIMAL FOOD INTAKE

What kinds and quantities of food give us greatest longevity, taking into account how 'The Base of Our Environment' can affect a clean body in the ?

Optimal Food Intake is the ideal equation of quality and quantity of food for greatest longevity, in a given environment.

Dr. Norman Walker's Diet is the best model I have found to illustrate *The Optimal Food Intake.* If you recall, he is reported to have lived well past 100 on the very diet you are about to learn. (There is some controversy about the exact length of Dr. Walker's life. Regardless of how long he lived, I still consider his model of eating as The Optimal Food Intake.) Keep in mind that he lived in Prescott, Arizona, in an area where the environment was superior to average city air. Also, we cannot forget that over the years, our environment has deteriorated. If the deterioration continues at the same rate over the next 50 years, we will be living on an entirely different planet than Dr. Norman Walker experienced. Thus, adjustments to this blueprint may be appropriate depending on where you live and the general condition of our Earth. Hopefully, however, the modifications will be necessary because of vast improvements in our quality of living, and not the other way around.

Less is More

Most likely, this optimal food intake is far less quantity than your current diet. Reaching this Optimal Diet is best considered a long-term goal. It is recommended that you settle into your *Optimal Food Intake* gradually, over the course of many years. A slow but sure reduction in quantity will help your mind and body settle into change gently. Plus, there will be less likelihood of binge attacks and other eating disorders.

Pace Yourself

Eating less is the primary catalyst to becoming younger. Said another way, eating less is what makes us become younger! Ideally, you want to prolong this process of reducing your intake for as long as possible, so that you can enjoy the effects of becoming younger and maximize longevity. Reducing your quantity of food and jumping straight into an Optimal Food Intake would eliminate this window of opportunity to become younger. Instead, you would stabilize out at the Optimal Food Intake and then at some point be forced into the stage of slow aging on a Raw Food Diet. Additionally, you would become sensitive early on, limiting your margin for error and inconsistencies with kinds and quantities of food. Take your time and HAVE FUN!

In this case, slower is better to create a positive full-being experience, to continue becoming younger, maximize longevity, and keep the environmental threats at bay.

Longest Duration Of Life

Optimal Diet   **Environment Least Detrimental**

‒ ‒ ‒ ‒ ‒ ‒ ‒ ‒ ‒ ‒ ‒ ‒ ‒ **Optimal Food Intake** ‒ ‒ ‒ ‒ ‒ ‒ ‒ ‒ ‒ ‒ ‒ ‒ ‒

Myths

Every single person is an individual and there are over 1,000 variables going on in the human body at one time. By no means do I assume that everyone's diet should look the same. If someone is, for example, thriving on two meals a day, and they are instead told to eat many meals to suit their body type, this can actually be detrimental for them. People cannot be grouped so crudely. Each person is unique and food needs will change based on lifestyle and personality. For example, an extreme amount of emotional anxiety speeds up metabolism, possibly creating a need for more nourishment. This is not due to "body type", but stress management. Others medicate themselves with food all day, justifying their habit with reasons of blood type or even astrological sign.

Someone who thinks they have blood sugar issues may be told to eat six times a day. On this frequent feeding, they start to feel better, and assume their blood sugar normalized. Truly it all boils down to levels of toxicity. The endogenous poisons released during detox may cause shaking, fatigue and cravings. Constant eating stops this challenging detox and people feel more comfortable.

A drug addict, who snorts cocaine twice a day, becomes accustomed to his/her typical amount. If they cut back to once a day, withdrawal symptoms such as low energy, moodiness, and cravings for "a fix" will inevitably follow. This is not because their blood sugar went down. Do you see the inaccurate justification for what is really a system going through detox? With the help of a reliable alternative health practitioner, listen to your body and let it run its course for your healing.

As soon as you refill the stomach with food, THE ELIMINATION IS STOPPED and you feel better!
(Arnold Ehret: The Mucusless Diet Healing System, Pg. 156)

It Will Happen Naturally
The truth of the matter is that when someone is truly 100% Raw, as the years go on, they will naturally evolve to need less and less food. No matter what your gender, body type, or blood type, any individual can reach this proposed *Optimal Food Intake* over time, just as anyone can become a Liquidarian. My recommendation is not to go further or reduce your food quantity <u>below</u> this Optimal Diet, as the adverse conditions of the environment may affect your health in the long-run.

10
OPTIMAL HABITS

Shared Wisdom

We don't need to reinvent the wheel every time we wish to improve our situation. It is our nature as humans to learn from observing our personal experience AND observing the experience of others, good or bad. The other element to an optimal experience is the proper studying and gathering of facts. Success leaves clues.

I am 100% confident that *Raw Success* offers you the ultimate concepts for health and vital longevity. With that being said, however, I always encourage you to trust your *inner health practitioner*, for only you can know what is best for you from moment to moment. The perfect plan for you is to take in the information and foods that intuitively feel great.

In the spirit of sharing wisdom, let us continue to learn from the Centenarian himself.

Dr. Norman Walker lived 118 years.
What did he do right?

The Diet of a Centenarian

The Optimal Diet reflects the smaller portion requirement of an evolving 100% Raw Foodist. In Walker's book, *Vegetarian Guide to Diet and Salad,* he offers 70 different salad combinations – his personal favorites. The fat quantity per meal never exceeds **2 tablespoons**

of nuts and **½ an avocado**; often, it is just the ½ **avocado.** In addition to fat, the salads contain a maximum of ½ **a cup of vegetables** (consisting of a few tablespoons each of different chopped veggies) and/or **0-1 cup of fruit.**

Here is an example of one of Walker's pocket-sized salads:

Lettuce, ¼ head crisp and fresh	*- Coarsely chopped*
Celery, 2 or 3 stalks	*- Finely chopped*
Cucumber, ½ large (do not peel)	*- Finely grated*
Parsley, 1 tablespoonful	*- Finely minced*
Onions, 3 or 4 small green	*- Finely chopped*
Asparagus 2 or 3 stalks,	*- Finely chopped*
* fresh and crisp*	
Cauliflower, 2 teaspoonfuls	*- Finely grated*
Beets, 2 medium sized, fresh, young	*- Finely grated*
Peas, fresh tender green,	*- Use whole*
* 1 or 2 tablespoonfuls*	
Avocado, ½ medium sized	
Lettuce Leaves	

Arrange crisp leaves of lettuce on dinner plate and place the above vegetables in layers, each in the rotation given, sprinkling the whole green peas over the top of the beets and garnishing with the strips of avocado.

(Norman Walker: The Vegetarian Guide to Diet & Salad, Pg. 50-51)

As you can see, Dr. Walker always ate well under a quart of food and "sensible" amounts of fat and fruit. At my current level of evolution, his salads always leave me hungry, so I make them larger. I am in no rush to get to a position where I eat the same quantities as he did, because I see the brilliance behind taking things slowly.

Overeating

Dr. Walker seemingly never overate. *"Overloading the stomach taxes every function of the body and shortens life. The capacity of an average stomach is equivalent to about one quart, or four cups. Overindulging the right kind of foods, even in correct combinations, still puts tremendous stress on our organs". (*Norman Walker: Diet & Salad, Pg. 82) Additionally, eating an excessive amount stretches the stomach and you will crave more food the following day.

Chewing

Norman Walker also advocated and enjoyed the experience of *Fletcherism*. Fletcherism is the practice of chewing each bite of food until, as liquid, is goes down the throat without consciously needing to swallow. Generally it requires a minimum of 32 bites, depending on what you are eating. Chewing this thoroughly is even better for your health than having blended food meals (which are excellent) because the foods get more of a chance to mix with our enzyme-rich saliva.

Imagine yourself on a desert island, with only small rations of food. Likely, you would chew well to prolong the experience and garner all the nutrients you can. Instinctively, we know that meticulous chewing is the most effective way to nourish. The less one eats, the easier it is to Fletcherize, to the point where it is almost automatic.

Overlapping

From what I have been able to ascertain through my studies, Dr. Walker ate once or twice a day, plus juicing, and never snacked between meals. Unless the veggie juice was a part of his meal, he would make sure that his entire previous meal was digested before juicing again. It is an important practice to avoid the damage from fermentation, putrefication and partial digestion, which result from overlapping meals. Whenever possible, wait until the stomach is completely empty before intaking more juice or solids.

Variety

Dr. Walker made sure to get a wide variety of Raw Foods. Each one of Walker's unique salad recipes includes exciting combinations of different vegetables, fruits, nuts and seeds. His juicing selection was also very mosaic, to ensure a full spectrum of elements and minerals from our vast veggie kingdom. He made sure to only eat organic produce, void of pesticides and high in nutrients. It was a joy for Norman to grow much of the produce himself.

Daily Routine

Upon rising, Dr. Walker would drink a glass of hot water with lemon to flush the liver and kidneys. After 15-30 minutes, he would have a glass of orange juice to provide an ample supply of Vitamin C to assist in the regeneration of his connective tissue. Vitamin C is not produced or manufactured by the body; it must be obtained from food. Allowing another 15-30 minutes, he would then drink his first glass of fresh vegetable juice. That was Norman's entire breakfast. Generally he ate one or two solid meals during the day, consisting of one of his small salads or no more than a pound of fresh fruit.

As you can see, his quantities were small compared to the average eater. Consistent and disciplined in his routine, he ate to satisfy his bodily need and ate enough so that the environment was not a threat. He lived in the countryside. If Norman lived in the heart of a city, this diet would have needed to be adjusted to protect himself against the environment and he most likely would not have lived as long.

Concentrated Foods - Precious Nuts, Seeds, and Sprouts

Furthermore, Norman Walker stresses the importance of eating a small amount of seeds and sprouts every day, plus a few handfuls of nuts each week. A good rule of thumb is to not exceed one handful of nuts per day. Sometimes Dr. Walker ate a small handful of nuts alone or with raisins or figs as his lunch. Nuts are best either ground, soaked overnight, or soaked and dehydrated. Dehydrating prevents nuts from molding and allows for extended shelf life. Almonds, filberts (hazelnuts), and pumpkin seeds are an ideal choice for us because of their rich nutrient profile and low acid-forming properties.

Small amounts of nuts and seeds are a Raw Food Eater's most valuable source of concentrated fats and proteins. These tiny powerhouses are stuffed with nutrition. As you know, an entire plant grows from a single seed. After seeds are soaked, you can see them begin to sprout. In addition to possessing the same amount of nutrients as a full-grown plant or tree, the seed is obviously pulsing with *Life*. Besides nutrients, proteins, and fats, concentrated foods are key to long-term *Raw Success* because they hold the body back from evolving too far, too fast.

Remember, the less we use our digestive tract – by eating less and cutting out concentrated foods – the more we evolve and exist at a higher vibration. Our dense polluted Earth and daily stresses can be harmful to our sensitivity and ultimately limit vital longevity.

Raw Goat Products

Norman Walker was 100% Raw, but not vegan. His recipes often include minimal amounts of cheese from unheated, unpasteurized goat milk. A few of his salad recipes use **two ounces of Raw goat's milk cottage cheese.** Raw goat milk products are somewhat mucus-forming but can be handled in small quantities. Goat's milk cottage cheese, swiss cheese, and sour cream are preferred, as these are the least acid-forming. Raw goat's milk products are high in calcium, fluorine, and thiamine. Calcium is building for the bones and teeth, fluorine does wonders for our nails, blood, hair and skin, and *thiamine is one of the most important of the B-complex vitamins, involved in all of life's vital processes from birth to the grave. Raw goat's milk abounds with thiamine. *(*Norman Walker: Fresh Vegetable & Fruit Juices, Pg. 69)* Dr. Norman Walker kept his own goats to provide him with this valuable form of *varied* nourishment.

After seven years being Raw, I have never eaten goat products. From a strict vegan platform, there are veggies you can consume that have plenty of calcium and fluorine. I personally take a B-12/B-6 supplement, which is listed in the Resource Guide.

Mineral Supplements

Norman Walker was a fiery advocate for the complete range of trace elements (minerals). He supplemented his diet of Raw Foods and juices with:

- Homeopathic zinc
- ¼ of a teaspoon of alfalfa powder when fresh was not available to juice
- Dulse – in a bowl on the table, to grab from at every meal
- Kelp – in a shaker on the table
- Ocean seawater (not water from inland seas or lakes) – a few drops in liquids, salads, and other food

Dr. Norman Walker writes scientifically and personally about the benefits of Ocean seawater, a resource we surely don't want to miss:

All the mineral and chemical elements in Sea Water are already in colloidal or liquid form, and in their inherent state. In fact, they are so naturally concentrated that it requires only a minimal amount, actually a matter of a reasonably small number of drops, to vitalize and energize a whole tumbler full of fruit or vegetable juices.

As a matter of fact, we always keep a pint bottle of Catalina Sea Water (which we buy at the health food store) in our kitchen and add a few drops from it to every beverage, even to pure straight water when we drink it, and to our salads and other food. In this way we feel confident that we are getting our quota of trace elements into our system every day.

Of all the 59 trace elements, we have found that Zinc is involved in nearly every function and activity of the human anatomy.

(Norman Walker: The Natural Way to Vibrant Health, Pg. 98-99)

Dr. Norman Walker used homeopathic zinc. These days we have more options available to us, and I prefer to take zinc in its angstrom mineral form. Angstrom plant minerals are up to one million times smaller than colloidal minerals (contained in most supplements on the market), making them virtually 100% bio-available, instantly! Rather than large nutrients floating around the bloodstream, angstrom minerals are small enough to be absorbed into the cells and used immediately.

For seawater, I use *OceanGrown's Ocean Solution*, from Florida. At this point the company recommends this product for growing vegetation only, but I use it as Dr. Walker did. The Catalina Sea Water he speaks about is available on-line and in stores. After some thorough research, however, I discovered that the companies add other ingredients to the mixture, so I have yet to find a recommendable brand. My salads also often include copious amounts of dulse and kelp, as they are high in certain minerals from the ocean that are not available from common vegetables.

Here is another excerpt from Norman Walker about obtaining all the trace elements. He writes that he and his wife tried to eat at least 2-3 of the following foods every day:

> *Lack or unbalance of any one or more of these elements has a direct bearing on the health and sickness that assails humanity. It is of vital importance that they be constantly kept replenished and in balance in the system. Foods high in all the elements are alfalfa, beets, cabbage, capsicum, carrots, cucumbers, leaf dulse, filberts, jersualem artichokes, kelp, mung beans, olives, papayas, pine nuts, pumpkin seeds and water cress. Of course, all other foods not listed here do contain trace elements, but usually in lesser quantities so that by eating plenty of all available fresh Raw vegetables and fruits, and particularly drinking their juices, we can be fairly certain that we are getting our complement of the trace and other elements which the system requires.*
>
> *(Norman Walker: The Vegetarian Guide to Diet & Salad, Pg. 9)*

Systematic Under-Eating For Long-Term Success

In *Raw Spirit*, I wrote about how systematic under-eating means consuming just enough food to maintain life, while making sure to get all the nutrients your body needs. It is a road to ultimate regeneration, the key to longevity. When someone is systematically under-eating, like Dr. Norman Walker did, they finish their meal with a slight sensation of hunger.

When you eat small amounts of food, absorption is at its best. The body can utilize every last bit of a small meal if one is in the habit of systematic under-eating. Another plus is that we automatically tend to chew small meals more thoroughly, and this practice releases more of the nutrients and results in better digestion.

Many Raw Foodists overeat and/or eat all day long, seven days a week. In the beginning, they can get away with this type of behavior because their new Raw Lifestyle is such a vast improvement from their previous diet. However, going Raw is like getting into the world's fastest jet plane. Destination: Ultimate Health.

Quickly the body cleanses, evolves and stabilizes out on a Raw Diet. If excessive eating habits still persist, symptoms may appear such as Candida, skin blemishes, dental trouble, bloating, fatigue, and so on.

To offset the effects of poor Raw eating, it is common for some Raw Foodists to use Colon Hydrotherapy and consume a lot of enzymes. Although they may experience relief initially, there is a catch. Colon Hydrotherapy and enzymes are likely the most powerful cleansing tools on the planet. They catapult health to the next level and speed up our body's evolution, ultimately resulting in even less margin for error, and increased symptoms if poor eating habits continue.

It is NOT an easy task for most people to stop an eating habit. It can feel extremely painful emotionally. However, to gain the full benefit of the 100% Raw Food Diet, and to live past the century mark, we must seek to shift our eating habits.

11
FRUIT, FAT AND FERMENTATION

Is it dangerous to consume too much of a certain food?
If done consistently over a long period of time, you betcha!
Especially on a diet of Raw Foods.

Too Much Fruit!

Some long-term 100% Raw Foodists run into troubles from eating an excessive amount of fruit. Dr. Bisci has seen numerous disheartening cases of people living primarily on fruit for many years. These unfortunate individuals experience decaying teeth, hair loss, nutritional deficiencies and a host of other maladies. **We have never seen anyone succeed in the long-run on a diet consisting primarily of fruit.** The Raw Pioneers who chose this type of diet did not do well.

I want to discuss the consequences of *fermentation,* in regards to our fruit and sugar intake. To make this point clearer, it is important for you to understand that sugar is a key ingredient for fermentation. Fermentation is the chemical reaction which occurs when glucose (sugar) converts to carbon dioxide and energy (ATP). Carbon dioxide is irritating to our cells and tissues, when not eliminated. *{If you recall from the description above about how we consume air, our blood eliminates carbon dioxide waste as quickly as possible, and exchanges it for fresh oxygen.}*

Everything we eat breaks down to glucose (sugar) so

it can be converted into energy (ATP) by the cells of our body. The amount of sugar present in this conversion process determines the amount of fermentation. Eating straight sweet fruit causes more fermentation than eating fat due to the amount of sugar present. Fat *slowly* converts into glucose, giving us a steady supply of energy, while eating sugar fruit is like taking a straight shot of whiskey.

We can handle a certain amount of natural sugar without a problem. In fact, fruits and natural sugars, in reasonable quantity, have a soothing, alkalizing effect on the body. However, if we frequently eat sweet fruit in massive quantities, the resulting levels of fermentation create a highly *acidic* condition in the body from all the carbon dioxide – gaseous acidic waste – being produced.

I have also found that those who eat mostly fruit typically do not choose to consume concentrated foods such as nuts and seeds. Eliminating these dense foods from the diet moves one even closer to a fasting state, causing increased cellular detox, which adds to the already excessive fermentation from over-consuming fruit.

Increased detox + fermentation from excess sugar = tremendous acidic condition

Remember, the Raw Diet is a Life-Long Fast and the detox will always be there to a certain extent. In the long-run, **an acid body starts to leach alkaline salts from its skeletal frame to combat the over-acidic condition.** This is one of the reasons long-term Fruitarians and many Raw Foodists have problems with their teeth.

Some think simply adding more greens to their diet will fix the problem. True, adding greens helps to alkalize the body while at the same time providing extra precious minerals and nutrients. If someone adds greens, but continues to over-consume fruit, they may feel better initially. However, especially if they are not cleansing their colon, overeating fruit will inevitably catch up to them in the long-run even if they are eating more greens.

Please do not misunderstand. I LOVE FRUIT! **I eat fruit every day. It is an integral, enjoyable, nourishing part of my diet.** On rare occasions I will even overeat a favorite fruit that lures me in. However, that is an exception and only lasts one meal. If I were to overeat fruit twice that day or the following day, I would suffer the effects tenfold. It's what you do MOST of the time that really counts, rather than the little 'blips' here and there.

Fruit vs. Fat

I would rather see someone overdoing fat than fruit. This does not mean I advocate eating massive amounts of fat. Although less harmful than overeating fruit, for long-term success the ideal is to find balance in your intake of all the food groups.

If you truly become 100% Raw, over the years you will automatically evolve to need less food.

Seven years ago, I plunged into a 100% Raw Lifestyle overnight. After being on the typical American diet all my life, I was totally unaccustomed to the empty (yet not hungry) feeling in my stomach. I had a wild need to feel *full*. Thus, my evening ritual revolved around a HUGE salad that consisted of a LARGE head of romaine lettuce, 10 cut up heirloom tomatoes, over an ounce of dulse, a handful of sprouts, olives and 3 ENORMOUS avocados from the California Farmers' Market. I ate this gigantic salad every night for more than THREE YEARS! This is how I survived the transition! That large salad was one of the tools I needed for my success on the 100% Raw Diet. Gradually, I evolved and by year five or six I never ate more than one avocado in any one day and my salads were miniature in comparison.

In *Raw Spirit* I share the story of a man who went 100% Raw, lost 50 pounds and was experiencing a miraculous recovery from degenerative disease. During the gathering at which we met, he declared to our group that he ate a jar of almond butter every day, got knocked out from all the fat and protein, and then fell asleep. In spite of his almond butter habit, this man was losing massive amounts of excess weight and healing his body. I was thrilled to hear the advice given to him: "You are doing great! Keep up the good work. Who cares if you eat a jar of almond butter a day and fall asleep? Eventually that impulse will be gone. For now, eat all the almond butter you want." Just as I am not eating three large avocados anymore, I would guarantee that he is not still eating that daily jar of almond butter.

I heard David 'Avocado' Wolfe once say that he used to eat nine avocados a day when he first became Raw. Now I'm sure he is not able to handle anywhere near that volume.

For ultimate long-term success, we do not want large amounts of fat in our daily diet. If you are eating large amounts of fat at this time and choose to cut back, **be careful to avoid a drastic increase in your quantities of fruit intake instead,** for that will inevitably cause complications. If you look at the quantities of fat and fruit that Dr. Norman Walker ate, you will notice that he routinely consumed a small amount of each in his meals. The Optimal Diet is an ideal balance of fat and fruit. Be sensible, trust yourself, and learn from the successes and pit-falls of others.

12
ADDITIONAL SUPPORT
How can I make sure I'm getting all my body needs?
Juice, Supplement and Cleanse.

Other Beneficial Supplements

It is rare to find a 100% Raw Foodist whose habits are comparable to Dr. Walker – country home, small well-chewed infrequent meals, fresh vegetable juicing, and colon cleansing. The supplements he took and recommended were sufficient for a near "perfect" diet and lifestyle, creating near-perfect nutrient absorption. If you commit to the diet and habits of Dr. Walker, I believe his recommendations are all you need, once your body has stabilized out. However, we are not all ready or willing to take on that standard of living. For many of us, it is wise to have extra support.

The following supplements were not on Dr. Walker's list, but they are certainly on mine!

Enzymes

Dr. Norman Walker praises the miraculous benefits of the enzymes in Raw Food. Back in his day, enzyme supplements did not yet exist. I am convinced that had they been available, Dr. Walker would have valued them as he would a winning lottery ticket!

As precious as powdered gold, enzymes are extremely valuable for the Raw Foodist. Simply said, they prolong life! Although best known for their power as a digestive aid, their hidden potential far surpasses that function.

There are two types of enzymes produced by and in our body:

(1)   Metabolic enzymes – which we depend on for life
(2)   Digestive enzymes – to digest food

Metabolism is the total of all chemical changes that take place in a cell or an organism to produce energy and basic materials needed for important life processes. *Metabolic enzymes*, perfectly named, are involved in every process of the human body. In fact, even digestive enzymes start as metabolic enzymes. Besides our day-to-day life processes of build up and breakdown, these little powerhouses are catalysts that take an active role in repairing any damage done to our body through injury, stress, poor eating or lifestyle habits, environmental contaminants, and the passage of time.

Unfortunately, we don't have an unlimited supply of metabolic enzymes. We are born with a certain reserve of these petite miracles, and when this reserve runs out, our life ends. Our body does, to some extent, replenish metabolic enzymes, but the numbers used versus the numbers added still make them something to cherish.

When you take any type of enzyme, you are conserving your storehouse of metabolic enzymes. Enzymes taken with food, for example, save the metabolic enzymes that would have needed to be converted into digestive enzymes. Although Raw Food retains its natural enzymes, it is good to remember that within an hour of picking, a great percentage of the enzymes are lost. It's a sad affair to know that when we buy produce from the health food store, it has voyaged by truck (often many miles), and has likely been sitting on the shelf for days. Therefore, it is a life-prolonging practice to take digestive enzymes with meals made with such foods.

Enzymes taken on an *empty stomach* serve a remarkably different function than digestion. These enzymes are immediately directed to the metabolic processes of our bodies. There are experiments that involve coupling radioactive particles with ingested enzymes, allowing scientists to track the path of enzymes. Results prove that enzymes taken on an empty stomach do indeed assist the metabolic functions, including the miraculous repair of any damage sustained by the body. *Translation:* More Life – we age slower and have more energy!

Our bodies are designed in such a way that we do not have to consciously play a part in the trillions of actions taking place in the body. However, oftentimes, we are simply not aware of the effect our actions have, good or bad. If you take enzymes today, you may not notice any phenomenal immediate change. In the long-run, however, you will appreciate your enzyme-rich prolonged life. You could live a long and healthy life without ever taking enzymes. Yet, what could your life be like *with* them? I feel it is foolish to not use this powdered gold every day for the rest of our lives.

I personally take enzymes on an empty stomach 2-3 times a day. Dr. Fred Bisci's *Therapeutic Enzymes*, available in the Resource Guide of this book, is the most powerful and effective enzyme blend on the market. If you are interested in a more packaged over-the-counter product, Vitalzym® could be an alternative.

Coupled with an improved diet, Colon Hydrotherapy, and vegetable juicing, Dr. Bisci uses Therapeutic Enzymes to help heal people from degenerative disease. These extraordinary enzymes have the potential to dissolve cancerous tumors when taken on an empty stomach. This is because of their assistance to the metabolic processes of the body, which repair damage. I have personally witnessed the miraculous reversal of certain degenerative health conditions when Therapeutic Enzymes were used consistently in conjunction with an improved diet.

With all that being said, I must state here that nothing is a panacea, a cure-all. Optimal Health and healing is a many-layered process. I recommend the support of a professional alternative nutritionist to assist in the healing of degenerative diseases through adhering to a better diet, cleansing, vegetable juicing, and enzyme therapy.

Vitamin D

The sun is our most natural source of Vitamin D. For those who live far from the equator, in cold climates with little sunshine, I feel it is crucial to take a Vitamin D supplement. Dr. Bisci does not shy away from giving people hefty dosages of Vitamin D, if the person's condition would benefit. This is done under supervision.

Super Green Foods

We need GREENS! One of the greatest challenges we face as modern-day Raw Foodists is eating enough nutritious greens. Our salads would have to be gigantic to get an optimal amount of greens, and even then, green nutrients can be locked tightly within the dense fibers. A few savvy and frustrated individuals faced with this dilemma found a solution: Super Green Foods.

Green Food is generally a mixture of choice dried organic veggies, algae, dark leafy greens, and will sometimes include other beneficial ingredients such as enzymes, probiotics, etc. Norman Walker took ¼ of a teaspoon of straight mineral rich alfalfa Green Food powder whenever fresh alfalfa was not available to juice. His absorbability was at full potential and he needed very little. I personally consume tablespoons of Green Food most days, especially when my habits are not at their best. Super Green Foods serve as an effective safety precaution to ensure you are getting enough minerals and nourishment to your body.

Please note that Green Food is not a replacement for juicing. There are two main reasons: (1) Vegetable juicing is more alkalizing; in fact, it is the most alkalizing thing you can do for your body. (2) *Nutrients in liquid form* are most absorbable by the body. Green Food consists of solid particles, even when mixed in water. Simply stated, fresh is best. These Super Greens are definitely nutritionally potent, convenient, and a beneficial source of rare algaes and greens.

Vitamin B_{12}

I feel that everyone, whether on a 100% Raw Food Diet, Standard American Diet, or anything in between, would benefit tremendously from taking a supplemental B_{12} Vitamin. Research shows that low red blood cell count, Alzheimer's disease, as well as chronic fatigue syndrome may all be caused by a Vitamin B_{12} deficiency. The body needs this B vitamin to make blood cells and to maintain a healthy nervous system. It is an essential nutrient for vital longevity.

At their peak performance and efficiency, our bodies naturally produce Vitamin B_{12}. Dr. Walker was likely one of the rare individuals to accomplish this. Yet he still ate Raw unpasteurized goat's cheese, which has an abundance of B vitamins. In today's environment, I feel it is not worth taking the risk that your body will produce B_{12} on its own. It doesn't hurt to take a B_{12} supplement, and thankfully, we can all easily partake of this valuable resource.

Probiotics

Probiotics are another supplement that was not available in the days of Norman Walker. Another "Godsend", probiotics not only provide and support beneficial bacteria in our colon, they also clean up our system internally, which results in less gas. In my own life, I definitely appreciate this support.

Blood Tests

I recommend a CBC blood test once every two or three years. A CBC blood screening test can show your levels of iron, Vitamin B_{12} and folate. Keep in mind that the "healthy" levels for a 100% Raw Food Eater can slightly vary from those recommended for a cooked food eater. Sadly, many 100% Raw Foodists neglect this useful tool of blood testing. It is preferable to catch any deficiencies early, before the consequences deepen.

Watch Out

Two sneaky factors that can work against longevity are:

- Not keeping up with the detox by regular Colon Cleansing
- Deficiencies from lack of supplementation and juicing

If you fall into the trap of neglecting to take care of these two necessities, then you won't have to worry about being in Optimal Balance, because either the lack of nutrients or your own inner toxemia will undermine your efforts at longevity.

13
STEP 4: EXPLORING THE RABBIT HOLE
Where should I live?
That answer could greatly depend on what you eat.

Where Do You Live?

Dr. Norman Walker lived in the countryside, not a polluted city. His minimal diet suited him fine in the clean country air. He balanced his quantity of food and his environmental pressures, awarding him a vibrant, long life. In a city dwelling, on this same diet, the dense toxic Base of The Environment *{see Chapter 4}* would have shortened his life.

Longest Duration Of Life

Optimal Diet   **Environment Least Detrimental**

‒ ‒ ‒ ‒ ‒ ‒ ‒ ‒ ‒ ‒ ‒ ‒ ‒ **Optimal Food Intake** ‒ ‒ ‒ ‒ ‒ ‒ ‒ ‒ ‒ ‒ ‒ ‒

For long-term *Raw Success*, we must consider: *Location*. With the ever purifying body of a long-term Raw Vegan, living in a large city or neighboring polluted suburbs can definitely have an adverse effect on our health now and in the long-run. We do not all have to make a run for the Himalayas though. It is enough to find a little nook with good air quality, as close to the hub of city action as you desire. This will ensure that The Base of Your Environment doesn't get the best of you in the long-run. For example, I live 75 miles outside Los Angeles, under the uncontaminated skies of Ojai, CA.

Improving Your Diet

95% of those reading this book do not have to worry about "too clean a diet", unless you live in an extremely polluted environment. There are a few reasons for this. Most people I encounter are not 100% Raw. There is a big difference in the body of a person who is 100% Raw versus even 95% Raw. At 100% Raw, each improvement in diet causes an exponential raise in sensitivity. The further you go down the "rabbit hole" of eating better quality and less quantity of food, the more sensitive you become. Additionally, the mass majority of people who are 100% Raw, have not taken their diet even close to the optimal food intake recommended in this book. A high percentage of 100% Raw Vegans are in fact at the other extreme, it seems, continually eating throughout the day, seven days a week.

Consider also, the length of time one is Raw. Many reading this book are likely in their beginning few months, or have been Raw just one to three years. This is still the stage of detoxing previous years of poor eating, which is a massive project that can continue for over a decade, depending on your initial state of toxemia. For the long-term 100% Raw Foodist, as their quantities of food naturally reduce, the more careful they must be to balance their diet with The Base of Their Environment.

Generally, the rabbit hole of an improved diet looks like this:

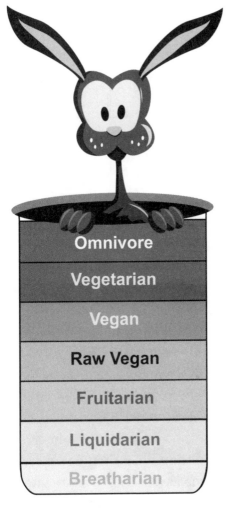

*!*When you eat less than the suggested optimal food intake for a Raw Vegan or if you go beyond the Raw Vegan lifestyle to a Fruitarian and so on, you are in the WARNING ZONE for long-term *Raw Success*. Sensitivity starts to increase *exponentially*.

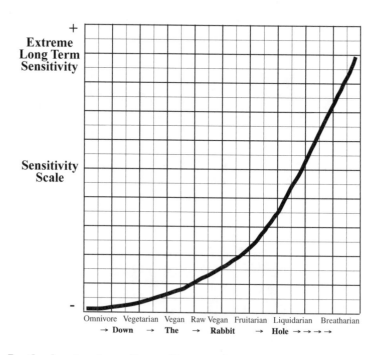

Omnivore	Vegetarian	Vegan	Raw Vegan	Fruitarian	Liquidarian	Breatharian
→ **Down**	→	**The**	→	**Rabbit**	→	**Hole** → → → →

In the beginning of any dietary change, most people have masses of energy and do pleasingly well. Vitality and life increase profoundly! However, because of today's environmental condition, we must be cautious. The above graph illustrates that the further you take your diet down the rabbit hole, the more sensitive you become. Once again, it is paradoxical that those in a weakened condition, who are eating a less than ideal diet, can tolerate and endure adverse conditions longer than a more vital body.

In the long-run, the polluted external Base of Our Environment may start to deteriorate health in someone who is extremely sensitive, because of his or her pristine inner condition. A Liquidarian or Breatharian would be unlikely to thrive in Los Angeles. A 100% Raw Food Eater may be able to outlive and out-energize many cooked food eaters, but for long-term *Raw Success* way past the century mark, there is a cost – we must eventually choose an environment conducive to such a "Heavenly" lifestyle.

Extreme Dieting

*Why would someone continue to travel further
down the rabbit hole?*
Why choose to eat less and less?
The benefits.

Every time dietary improvement is made, one feels and becomes younger, healthier, more vital. Spiritually, the effects can be unimaginable. In *Raw Spirit*, I wrote about my own spiritual rebirth. Whenever I try to explain my energetic and spiritual transformation to a mainstream thinker, it seems they usually cannot fathom, cannot relate to the depth of connection that I experience on a daily basis. When one maintains an improved diet and does appropriate internal cleansing, the body becomes a more in-tune receiver of spiritual vibrations. Spiritual transformation is enhanced the less food one eats, or the farther down the "rabbit hole" one travels.

Just as most people don't seem to identify with my spiritual life, I cannot accurately imagine the spiritual state of a successful long-term Liquidarian, who does appropriate internal cleansing. Through my journey, I have met *Experimenters*, those who have taken the leap to "extreme pure dieting" – taking in miniscule amounts of food for a considerable amount of time. Here is one story from an Experimenter: If a woman walked in the room without making a sound, he could sense they had entered and even knew if they were in their menses or not. The energetic sensory abilities these extreme dieters enjoy are way beyond what I can identify with. My own short fasts and juice fasting merely scratch the surface.

In your own process of exploration, please, please keep in mind the risk these extreme pure dieters have undertaken. In the long-run there is serious danger of shock from any inconsistencies in amount or quality of foods, and from the pollution in the environment. Most likely these individuals will suffer complications in the long-run. Yet, some people may make the choice for a more energetic vibratory life with a higher potential for spiritual experience, even at the expense of their life span.

Back up the Rabbit Hole

My diet is consistent and fairly pure, making me "sensitive" compared to the average individual. The Breatharian or Liquidarian is even more susceptible than I. To go back up the rabbit hole optimally, one must return very slowly. The further down you travel, the more carefully you must ascend.

If I were to return to a Standard American Diet, it would not be as simple as hopping in my car and going to stand in line at the local burger joint. As I have said before, I am 98% sure that shocking my system with a greasy hamburger would put me in the hospital. A long-term Liquidarian or Breatharian, who is consuming miniscule amounts of nutrition and wants to return to solid foods, even 100% Raw Food, would be faced with an even larger obstacle than I would have going back to a cooked food diet.

14
STEP 5: EMOTIONAL AND SPIRITUAL HEALTH

Does adopting a Raw Lifestyle bring up suppressed emotions?
Definitely. You are in for quite a ride!

The Secret Ingredient

Emotional and spiritual health is THE MOST important step to long-term Raw Success. Upon choosing a 100% Raw Diet, you are automatically thrown into these more subtle realms of life. The body vibrates with increased spiritual energy. *{The section, The Science Behind It All, scientifically theorizes why a Raw body vibrates at such a significantly higher frequency.}*

Additionally, since cooked foods are not there to medicate the senses, any emotional and psychological issues bubble up to the surface. All those buried emotions of fear, sorrow, jealousy, and feelings of inferiority show up to be dealt with. Healing this requires awareness, direct attention, and likely some truthful expression.

It's my belief that the Top Two reasons an individual fails to sustain a 100% Raw Diet are:

1. Failure to do internal cleansing
2. Inability to handle the emotional and psychological trauma that arises

If you recall, when we experience negative emotions – anger, fear, jealousy, hatred – the adrenal glands produce adrenalin in excess. The potency of this adrenalin secretion is poisonous! A basic example is that when one is under tremendous stress, pimples often show up on the face and elsewhere. In this case, pimples are the extra toxins produced by stress that are trying to leave the body.

Similar to adrenalin, Joy is also very potent. Our emotional health and feelings of well-being have a direct affect on our health. We all know that *laughter is the best medicine*. Nowadays, it is common to hear a story about someone who cured his or her degenerative disease through an improved lifestyle and MORE laughter. When I have a laugh attack, my entire body feels regenerated and renewed.

Having All The Answers

On the topic of longevity and spiritual growth, as with any topic, I feel I am far from having all the answers.

> *"The more I learn, the more I realize I don't know."*
> ~ *Albert Einstein*

I think it is wise to assume that there is always more to discover. I am attempting to share the best of what I understand thus far, and we shall all continue to grow, as we give attention to our goals and dreams.

Awareness is the First Step

For long-term *Raw Success*, it is important that we accomplish the tremendous task of developing control over our emotions. Nervous tension is a common trait among humanity. How many times have you seen someone with bouncy legs, fidgety movements, and nubby fingernails? Negative pent up energies affect our enjoyment of life and relationships, not to mention our health and digestion. Not staying calm often causes indigestion, noxious gas, and releases corrosive hormones caused by stress. It is important to be as peaceful as you can, especially during meals, for optimal health.

There is a technique I find particularly beneficial for managing energy. *Meditation.* Meditation is putting your attention on a specific point. It could be a physical sensation such as wind blowing on your face or the experience of breathing in and out. It can be the sound of ocean waves or something subtle like feeling the emotional energies present in your body.

Meditation is tremendous support for dealing with the psychological and emotional issues that often rise to the surface when one transitions to a Raw Food Diet.

I took to meditation like I took to fresh figs. As the days and hours ticked on, I began to notice a pain, a feeling of misery in my being. The sensation was not typical physical pain like bruising, muscle injury, or getting punched in the stomach; it was *more subtle.* Instinctively I felt drawn to put my complete attention on the place of greatest distress. Continual focus and meditation on the predominant sensation reduced the discomfort, healed it, and evolved me spiritually, as well.

For me, there was often a lot of nervous tension and emotional pain in my solar plexus, the area just above the naval. I wondered if, by continually focusing on the solar plexus, I could gain control over these negative energies.

To my naïve surprise, I was not the first to discover this method. Norman Walker sheds some light on why the solar plexus technique is so effective:

> *The nerves are involved in every motion and action of the body. Also, they are the first to sound an alarm when there is anything whatever wrong in the system, no matter how apparently unimportant it may seem. For example, when we have been overworking we come home irritated. That irritation results in tying us into a knot, inside, usually the region of the solar plexus. This solar plexus is a mass of nerves and muscles. It is one of the first parts of the body to respond to conditions outside of ourselves that we allow to affect us. When we have learned to have complete control over our solar plexus, we will have progressed a long way towards helping us become younger.*
>
> *(Norman Walker: Become Younger, Pg. 57)*

Negative emotional energies have a direct effect on our health. They start as subtle energy and can eventually wreak havoc on our life in the areas of health, finances, relationships, and personal fulfillment. Awareness of this fact is the first step in the right direction.

Disturbing energies can be with us the entire day to one degree or another. Diligence is required to discover them in all their different forms and volumes. I often practice while driving, lying in bed, and as much as I can throughout the day. If we can find disturbances at *point easy*, when they are first rolling around in the solar plexus or other areas of the body, we can focus our attention on the predominant sensation, heal those energies, and minimize anything showing up in our external world experience.

The key to ease and success with this technique is **complete, unwavering focus.** For a period of time, you must have ridiculous willpower. Focus your awareness on the most predominant *subtle energetic sensation,* no matter what you start experiencing. Like a heat-seeking missile, find the different negative energies, while keeping outrageously SHARP awareness, every millisecond, even when heart-thumping FEAR bears its teeth, as you face these energies head on. It is easy to avoid and lose awareness. Once again, for a certain period of time you focus – !Moment!After!Moment! !Instant!After!Instant! – continuing to meditate, no matter what happens.

From the pulpit of personal experience, I will tell you this: It is extremely likely that if you go deep into this kind of meditation, you will have subtle experiences "not of this world".

The more you can hone your ability to focus, the easier it is to find these negative energies floating around in your being and transform them, through the power of attention.

Think of meditation as a profoundly effective method of prevention. If I can prevent the negative energy from reaching *point crisis,* I conserve life force and ultimately live longer. It is consistently obvious to me that dynamic, positive energy accumulates when I meditate. All this extra life force is then directed to the well-being of my body. I feel continual awareness of the energies in our being is nothing less than essential for long-term *Raw Success.*

The Spiritual Gland

I think we would all agree that our body is energy, plain and simple. There are certain concentrations of energy inside our bodies, often called *chakras*. I am so grateful to Dr. Walker for providing logical scientific information about these energy centers. The solar plexus is one chakra he speaks about at length. There is also much attention given to our pineal gland energy center, otherwise known as the 6th chakra or "third eye".

In my book, *Raw Spirit*, I wrote about the opening of my third eye. I had been Raw six months and decided to do the psyllium/bentonite 7-day cleanse by Bernard Jensen. Immediately following the cleanse, I experienced such terrific sensations in my forehead that I was spellbound. I've since come to recognize these sensations as: Progress.

When addressing our emotional and spiritual health, it is important to understand that we are more than a dense physical body. I offer this information as a way to enhance our ability to live a long and fulfilled life. Awareness is the first step. Read on as Dr. Walker explains the scientific significance behind the third eye, that most fantastic pineal gland.

The pineal gland is undoubtedly the spiritual receptacle for life force emanating from the Cosmic Energy of the Universe. The pineal is such a small gland that scientists failed to assign any importance to it until the last 40 years, and even today the strict materialist does not appreciate its mental and spiritual significance.

The mental and spiritual influence of the pineal surpasses that of any other gland. It would almost seem as if this influence is directly connected to the relationship of the physical body of the individual and that mysterious and intangible part known as the soul.

The pineal gland is analogous to a radio antenna, receiving from the atmospheric environment the vital flow of cosmic energy acting like an electric current when it enters the body. Cosmic Energy is that infinite unfathomable power which permeates the entire universe holding the planets in their course and operating right into the very core of every atom in your body.

Like the current from one of the huge electric generating stations sending hundreds of thousands of volts through the wires to the 115 volt transformer near your home, so the universal cosmic energy enters the pineal • gland with inexpressibly high voltage which would virtually burn up the body if the body were not equipped with a transformer to lower that cosmic energy to the voltage consistent with the needs of the individual.

This cosmic energy transformer in the midbrain is known as the thalamus, a structure of a mass of gray cells and tissues in the midbrain which collects the energy from the pineal gland and lowers it and controls it to conform to the physical, mental and spiritual development and needs of the individual. Many people who understand this procedure classify the pineal gland as the spiritual gland in man.

(Norman Walker: Vibrant Health, Pg. 74)

15
WATER

What is the best water I can drink?
Distilled water and water distilled by nature, a.k.a. juice.

The Great Divide

Arenas of health are often split by passionate opinions from various "experts" and laymen. The topic of WATER has not been spared from this division; there is no unified agreement about which kind is best. The only water that is *only water* (i.e. *only* H_2O), void of everything else, is distilled. I don't trust anything else for my health.

If just one particle a day from non-distilled water remains in my body, the accumulation after 1000 days - under four years - would be shocking. Now imagine a lifetime of drinking lime-heavy spring water. Pounds and pounds of inorganic minerals would enter your system before they were hopefully eliminated.

Tap and spring waters are full of minerals from the Earth, soil, and rocks, plus various Man-added chemicals. These are classified as *inorganic minerals*. They do us no good because they are not *organic minerals* – minerals derived directly from plant life. Our cells reject them and these unusable elements are stored in the tissues, organs and arteries, hindering the functions of our body.

Distilled water has gotten flack from several professionals, claiming this mineral-void water *leaches* minerals from our body, causing deficiency and bone loss.

I am absolutely convinced this is a falsehood. When we drink distilled water, tests show there is mineral sediment in our urine. It is understandable to assume that we are being robbed of our precious organic minerals. In reality though, distilled water acts as a magnet, drawing to itself any inorganic minerals discarded by our cells and transporting them to the kidneys for elimination. The presence of these minerals in our urine is proof that we should have been drinking distilled water our entire lives, not avoiding it.

According to Norman Walker:

There is neither water nor any other liquid which can "*leach" minerals out of the cells and tissues of the body, once such minerals, as organic elements, have become an integral part of the body. It is only inorganic minerals rejected by the cells and tissues of the body which, if not evacuated, can cause arterial obstructions and even more serious damage. These are the minerals which must be removed and which distilled water is able to collect.

(Norman Walker: Water Can Undermine Your Health, Pg. 5)

*Our body's storehouse of precious organic minerals is used in daily living and must be replenished from various Raw Foods, juices, and supplements. Please do not confuse this need for replenishment as the body leaching out minerals. The two are vastly different.

Vegetable juices are made of the highest quality distilled water we could ever consume, plus they possess the perfect mineral balance. **Vegetable juice is water distilled by nature.** To ensure enough minerals for my body, I drink a sufficient amount of vegetable juice daily. In addition to juices, I drink at least two quarts of distilled water a day.

I add a drop or two of *Ocean Grown* to my water, as well as to my vegetable and fruit juices. The food available commercially to us today is not as nutritious or mineral dense as it was centuries ago, mainly due to topsoil depletion. I know that adding a bit of the seawater to my juice makes a world of difference. Lastly, I make sure to get plenty of seaweed in my daily diet.

16
A NOTE ABOUT: EXERCISE, REST, SLEEP, & MORE

If I'm eating all the best foods, isn't that enough for vibrant health?
Optimal Health requires more from you, but it gives back tenfold.

The Basics

There is more to most things than meets the eye. There are many spokes to a wheel. I created Raw Success to concentrate on the hub of vital longevity: ***An Optimal Diet in balance with our environment.*** Admittedly, this is a strong, yet single ingredient for the recipe of a long, healthy, happy life.

I believe that some other key ingredients are as follows:

The will to enjoy life! Having the will to live gives us tremendous vitality; it is difficult to even grasp the tremendous impact our desire to enjoy living has on our health. Think of waking up smiling, simply because we are overjoyed to be alive! It is also extremely important to get sufficient sleep, sunshine, and to exercise at least 30 minutes a day. Frequent ejaculation can also have an adverse effect on male health in the long-run. I go into detail about the effects of ejaculation in *Raw Spirit*.

These are the undeniable basics. The media and our tendency toward inertia seem to encourage us to shortcut these fundamentals, but the results are all too predictable: shorter life span and compromised well-being.

17
MY RAW PATH

Can I learn from someone else's journey?
**What moves and inspires you is no
longer just someone else's experience,
it is now yours as well.**

Home Sweet Home

As I write this, 84 months have come and gone since
I became 100% Raw Vegan. After my first year being
Raw, the air quality where I was living in New York
City was unbearable. Some research and traveling led
my sensitive lungs to a small town in Southern California, called Ojai. It has the best air quality I have found
within driving distance of my family.

Living somewhere with above average air quality, such
as my hometown, I feel is adequate for the long-run. At
some point in the distant future, I may desire to move
to an even cleaner environment for ultimate long-term
Raw Success, but it's not absolutely necessary. I do love
the feeling of living in the cleanest air possible though,
so I may be quite tempted. Pristine air is electric! In
clean environments, I feel my body evolving to become
a more in-tune vibrational machine.

What I Eat

*Here I will outline my typical daily meals
in the hope of helping you discover your own optimal path.*

Currently, I eat two meals a day without snacking, and drink a minimum of two 16 oz. vegetable juices. 95% of my juices contain dark leafy greens like spinach, romaine, turnip and radish greens, fenugreek, dandelion, or whatever I can find that is green. I love juicing wild greens that I just picked from the ground – I can feel their vitality tenfold! At some point, I am sure that I will have a greenhouse and/or garden to grow my own produce.

First thing in the morning I squeeze fresh lemon juice into a large glass of hot water. 15 to 30 minutes later I have an 8 oz. glass of fresh squeezed orange or grapefruit juice. 15 to 30 minutes following that I have my first green vegetable juice. Lemon water, citrus juice, and veggie juice - that is my standard breakfast.

Lunch is anytime between 11:00 and 2:00. Generally this amounts to a couple of pieces of fruit such as mashed bananas, mixed with a small amount of dried fruit, ½ a teaspoon of Celtic sea salt, and 4 to 6 tablespoons of seeds and nuts. Lately I have been an active guy – lifting heavy weights and running – so my quantity of seeds and nuts has increased. A few hours after lunch, I enjoy my second green juice.

In the evening, I usually have a salad with **1 large avocado.** Sometimes I'll include a small amount of additional fat such as **4 olives or a tablespoon of seeds.** The rest of my salad consists of about **three cups of vegetables with no fruit.**

That is the entire daily menu. Rarely, I'll indulge in a Raw restaurant or gorge myself on durian *(my Raw kryptonite, I just can't stop eating it!).*

Two meals a day has been my routine for the last seven years. Only the quantity of food in my meals has fluctuated. For the first few years, my evening salads had **2 to 3 BIG avocados.** Now my body bucks if I go over **1 ¼ avocado.** In the long-run I plan to eat smaller amounts of everything, similar to Dr. Walker. He usually had only ½ **an avocado** in his salad. Also, he only used ½ **a cup of vegetables** (compared to my 3 cups) with a **small amount of fruit.** If I combined fruit with my size meal, the food combination of fat and fruit may get the better of me. If I decreased my quantities, like the recipes from Norman Walker, the combinations would be very manageable.

Quantity

There are three reasons why I am not jumping on the Norman Walker bandwagon just yet:

#1 – Inevitably, I will become more sensitive as the years go by. The cleaner we become, the less room there is for error. I am a young guy who enjoys food and I do not want to limit myself more than I have already.

#2 – Obviously, I am passionate about becoming younger AND staying that way for as long as possible. If I were to jump into a diet like Dr. Norman Walker's right now, I would lose my entire margin to become younger. Initially, I would experience the fountain of youth, until I quickly stabilized out. To become any younger from that point, I would need to again eat less food. Eating less than my Optimal Diet would eventually put me in jeopardy with my environment. Maybe in five decades I will choose to live in a pristine environment and move further down the rabbit hole. For now, I would rather improve my diet slowly to extend my enjoyment of becoming younger.

#3 – Lastly, a gradual process of changing my diet will make for an easy psychological and emotional journey. I am no stranger to the jolt of extreme change – overnight I went from the SAD diet to 100% Raw Food! Going to the next level with anything in life takes a bit of adjustment. Stepping forward gradually can increase the chance for permanent, sustainable change. There is no doubt in my mind that at some point I will arrive at the place I aspire to be.

Having said all that however, it is true that if I chose to adopt an Optimal Diet right now, I would age slower and possibly increase my lifespan. But I would have to be spectacularly careful in the long-run with inconsistencies and the environment I choose to reside in.

Supplements
In addition to organic Raw Foods and a wide variety of fresh vegetable juices, I take the following supplements:

Angstrom Mineral Zinc – Zinc is the one mineral involved in almost every function and activity of the human machine. I don't feel that it is possible to intake a sufficient amount of zinc from food.

B-12, B-6, Folic Acid (all in one tablet) – To ensure I am getting a sufficient amount of the B vitamins.

Enzymes – To help digest food and conserve metabolic enzymes, which repair damage done to the body.

Probiotics – Reduce intestinal gas and provide beneficial bacteria for the colon.

Green Food – Dried vegetable juices. I enjoy alfalfa powder and an exciting variety of Green Foods, especially while traveling, as juicing can be impractical in some cases.

OceanGrown Seawater – For minerals. I add a drop or two in my vegetable juices, distilled water, and sometimes I remember to add seawater to my salads.

Vitamin D – I recommend this supplement to people who live in northern regions that lack consistent sunshine. Where I live, sunny days are in abundance. For those who need more however, Vitamin D is an important supplement to include.

Organic Variety

The single word *"Variety"* is foremost in my mind every time I go shopping at the Farmers' Market. I'm convinced that eating and juicing a wide range of fruits and vegetables makes my body smile, which translates to me smiling more. My salads always have a little chunk of unusual veggie or leaves of some exotic lettuce. For juice, I use the combinations laid out by Norman Walker. To that I usually add small amounts of new greens, roots, or veggies. Pulling nutrients from as many sources as possible, I make sure to eat a few seaweeds and an abundant assortment of seeds and nuts. I gather the majority of my food from organic farmers' markets around my hometown. 99% of my diet is organic produce. On occasion, if a non-organic mango whispers my name, I may indulge ...

Chewing
It is easy to overlook this most important ally to diges-tion and health.

On a cooked diet, and when I first switched to Raw, I wolfed down large bites, food barely touching my teeth. As my meals get smaller, my chewing gets better. Plus, Raw Foods seem to beg to be savored and chewed well. I do Fletcherize each delicious morsel most of the time if I am not in a rush. With Fletcherizing, I experience less gas, ridiculous off-the-charts energy, less need for food, and intense regeneration of my body. I've noticed that after being Raw for so long, it seems to be habitual and natural to chew well.

Internal Cleansing – Colon Hydrotherapy
The colon is the mysterious link between thriving and surviving. We will likely never fully comprehend all the benefits of internal cleansing on our quality of life. I believe it is irreplaceable as a healing tool.

I schedule a Colonic maybe three times a year, for deep cleansing and maintenance. When I first began my Raw adventures, I did Colonics frequently to clear out the major cesspool of cooked food eating. Then I switched to the at-home Colema Board®, which I used bi-weekly or monthly to keep up with the waste being eliminated, as my cells kept dumping years of toxicity into my system for elimination.

Now, I am pleased to share with you my latest dis-covery: the 6-quart Enema bag! Our colon can hold 4-6 quarts of water, depending on the individual. Traditional Enema bags hold 2-quarts of water, which is less effective for cleansing, as it only clears the lower colon. With some practice, you can do very effective cleansing for your entire bowel with the larger bag.

Whenever I feel sluggish, I do a 6-quart Enema. I usually fill and expel twice, using at most 4 of the 6-quarts for each fill. This process is so quick, effective, and portable – it feels like I struck gold!

The importance of cleansing the colon cannot be emphasized enough. I know it is one of the key reasons I am able to stay 100% Raw. As I've said, those who run into problems on the 100% Raw Diet often do not know why. Periodic colon cleansing would mean SUCCESS for 95% of these cases.

Colonic Irrigation Protocol

- Standard American Diet, not making improvements: 1 series every 6 months. *Typically, a series is two Colonics per week for five consecutive weeks.*
- [3]Intermediate Healthy Diet: *4 - 12 times a year*
- New Raw Vegan – up to 6 months Raw: *2 - 4 times a month*
- 6 months - 1 year Raw: *minimum once a month*
- 1- 3 years Raw: *minimum once a month*
- 3 years Raw and beyond: *minimum once a month*

Extra Colonics or high Enemas are helpful during healing crises, withdrawal, constipation, or intense detox symptoms.

---

[3] The Intermediate Diet is a protocol that Dr. Fred Bisci gives to most of his clients, which includes certain cooked grains and meats, in addition to Raw Foods. The complete diet can be found in my first book, *"Raw Spirit."*

Emotional and Spiritual Nutrition

An emotional and spiritual journey is not like a sentence – there is no period, no end. We have a natural human desire to keep experiencing more, and it is life's pleasure to offer us every opportunity.

My emotional and spiritual growth has been the finest reward of my Raw journey, thus far. There is of course much yet to unfold, in managing my emotions and negative energies. To continue growing, I meditate while driving, walking, and just simply as much as I can, whenever, wherever. Also, I use a release practice to move stuck energy, and occasionally shout at the top of my lungs in divine disgust! There is no time better spent.

My experience of this world grows more fantastic by the day.

Exercise

One of the "duhs" in life we just can't shortcut. Yes, I exercise – daily.

I love to exercise. Finding what I enjoy was a process, and I continue to vary my routine between weight lifting, running, biking, yoga, and walks. Currently I have a practice of lifting massive weight once a week, giving my body the entire rest of the week to recover. I find the results are impressive in terms of muscle mass and definition, but I am noticing that it also seems quite hard on the body. Yoga is a favorite of mine, and I usually do an hour session every morning, outside in the sun.

Running always gets the juices flowing. I feel like such a champion after I've gone a few miles and return home with a sweaty back and pounding heart. Currently, I run 2-3 miles, three or four times a week. I also highly value sleep and sunshine, and make sure to get plenty of each.

In Conclusion

"Raw for Life" is a popular expression. With what you have just learned, it is now possible to go *"Raw for Long Life."*

For that purpose, I offer *Raw Success* as your guide on the 100% Raw Vegan Diet. It is recommended that you study this book inside and out for the best understanding of all the variables already playing themselves out in your Raw experience. It took me many years of research, personal experimentation, and interviews with Raw Pioneers to fully integrate this information. Every bit of knowledge was like a seed that eventually blossomed into *Raw Success* – the truth, as complete and absolute as I am able to share it. For the best and longest life imaginable, I encourage you to also enjoy a thorough study of Dr. Norman Walker's books.

Gradually apply what you have learned.
There is no limit to what you can experience.
The rewards will far surpass what you can imagine.

APPENDIX A
WHAT YOU DON'T EAT

Healing is possible! Vibrant health is our birthright, and our responsibility.

I spend much of my time offering what I've learned, in the hope that it will inspire people to a happier, pain-free life. Many people ask me, "How do I become Raw?" First off, **you don't need to be 100% Raw to be healthy.** You can be very healthy on an intermediate transition diet without taking it to such an extreme as I have, with the 100% Raw Food Diet. I know how difficult it is. I am doing it!

So...**how does one begin the journey to better health?** There are a lot of diets out on the market today. I am sure you have heard about a few such as the Zone Diet, Macrobiotics Diet, South Beach Diet, Maker's Diet and others. Now I don't like to dismiss any of these programs because they can all produce positive results. I have personally witnessed people lose weight and heal from degenerative diseases after adopting these diet plans. There is one *common denominator* that allows these programs to succeed: they all require people to **leave out certain foods from their diets without exception!** Foods like refined sugar and processed starches are completely omitted. Because of this, a person's health improves considerably. The reason the 100% Raw Food Diet is the greatest diet in the world is because **you leave out everything that could make**

you ill and only keep in the most optimal, natural foods.

It is critically important to understand that what you leave out of your diet completely without exception is the way to ultimate health. What you don't eat is actually more important than what you *do* eat. **I don't care if you eat Raw Foods until you are blue in the face.** You are not going to fully heal unless you simultaneously eliminate the cause, which means omitting certain foods from your diet. I like to break foods down into the following five groups:

- Animal Protein
- Dairy
- Refined Sugar – Candy, Bakery items, Cake, Cookies
- Processed Starches – Bread, Pasta, Cereal
- Raw Vegan Foods – Vegetables, Fruits, Nuts, Seeds, and Sprouts

If what we leave out of our diet completely without exception is the way to ultimate health, then it makes sense to first eliminate the food groups that are most damaging to the body. **The two most damaging food groups are the refined sugars and processed starches. THAT IS THE SECRET!** That is what all those other diets do. Their plans require that you leave out the refined sugars and processed starches without exception! If you can do that one thing, you are on your way to ultimate health; you can live a very healthy life. I also recommend staying away from cooked red meat and pasteurized cows' dairy products. Those can all seriously undermine health.

I work with Dr. Fred Bisci, who has been on a 100% Raw Food Diet for over 40 years. He has a full-time Nutritional Practice and has helped thousands heal from deadly degenerative diseases. He uses an **Intermediate Healing Diet for those who don't want to go 100% Raw.** Many of the foods people enjoy are on this diet plan, including some tasty substitutes that offer a healthier option. He suggests Tinkyada Pasta, for example, which is a wheat and gluten free pasta, now available at most health food stores. Other 'intermediate' foods to enjoy are brown rice, beans, baked potato, whole grains, and sprouted grain bread.

There are certain rules in this Intermediate Diet, such as not mixing animal protein with starches and only eating 4-6 ounces of animal protein at most, every other day. If you only **ate the foods that are on this diet plan and nothing else, you could live to a very old, healthy age.** I knew a woman who tried the Intermediate Diet and healed herself from degenerative disease. She said that her arthritis went away after only two weeks. Fred gave permission for his Intermediate Healing Diet to be printed in my book *Raw Spirit*, available at www.Raw-Spirit.org. If you want to take this Intermediate Healing Diet to the next level, you can eliminate starches, such as Tinkyada Pasta and Brown Rice. If you are already 100% Raw, you do not need to follow this transitional diet. It would be like going backwards.

Many people I meet at my lectures tell me they are 70%, 80%, 90% Raw; this doesn't mean much to me. **They can eat 70% Raw, while the other 30% of the time they are eating pizza, soda, candy and cake.**

Now don't get me wrong. If you eat more Raw Foods, chances are your health will improve. But you are not going to do nearly as good as you could if you left certain foods out of your diet completely without exception. When you leave these certain foods out completely, without exception, this is when your body transforms, this is when your chemistry evolves, this is when your body becomes a more RECEPTIVE, IN-TUNE MACHINE TO SPIRITUAL ENERGY! This is not a matter of "religion". This is *physical!* Spiritual energy is something you can actually feel. My book *Raw Spirit* details the spiritual experiences I had when I became 100% Raw. Ever since then, my journey has just become richer.

Now let's talk about that second half of that phrase, "WITHOUT EXCEPTION". **If you continue to eat those foods, even if it is only every once in awhile, you don't give your body the freedom to take its healing to the next level.** Let's use an example of someone addicted to cocaine, who uses it every day. Let's say they quit completely, except once every two weeks. They will never detox the drugs at a cellular level. Why?

The following explanation applies to detoxing anything – from drugs, caffeine and nicotine, to processed sugars, wheat and dairy. Our cells are filled with waste from all the years of poor eating and they have expanded and grown to accommodate this waste. A certain amount of detoxification always takes place immediately, as soon as the quantity of drug or food is reduced. **However, the body holds onto the toxins stored at a deep cellular level, until the source of that particular**

toxin is stopped completely. To experience the next level of health, these buried poisons must be released. When you actually eliminate the drugs or foods completely, the toxins will leave your cells and now your body will have the freedom and the strength to take its healing to the next level.

Changing any habit can be challenging - physically, emotionally, and socially. I recommend taking it one food group at a time. The goal is to get rid of those refined sugars, processed starches, cooked red meats, and pasteurized cows' milk products. Also, it's best to not overdo animal protein or processed foods. On a good Intermediate Diet, you can be very healthy. You can also take it to the next level. **There is no rush. You can eliminate one food group at a time, taking months or years for each group.** Make it as slow of a process as feels good to you. Just try not to take steps backward. I recommend reading my book, *Raw Spirit* so that you can view Dr. Bisci's detailed Intermediate Diet. *Raw Spirit* is available at <u>www.RawSpirit.org</u>.

Your situation is not hopeless and you are not helpless. No single food supplement or medication can solve anyone's medical problem, ever. The body has natural remedial capabilities to heal itself, once you leave out the cause of disease. Diet is key. **What you leave out of your diet completely is what heals you.**

APPENDIX B
COMMON RAW SUCCESS
QUESTIONS & ANSWERS

1.   My husband eliminated flesh foods from his diet for 13 years. When he went back to eating meat, he felt great. Why didn't he experience the awful shock you speak about? Why instead did he feel even better than when he was Vegetarian?

There are thousands of variables occurring in the human organism at one time. If I was to guess, **I'd say your husband's colon is not clean.** Vegetarian diets usually contain processed foods that add to the layers of waste already on the colon walls. A clogged colon hinders the body's ability to take health to the next level. In this buffered condition, even sudden changes will not shock the body. **The meat most likely stimulated him and stopped any uncomfortable detox he may have been experiencing on a cleaner diet.**

Additionally, you have to keep in mind that the body raises to an entirely different echelon on a 100% Raw Vegan Diet. A totally Raw body evolves to a level of unparalleled sensitivity, the like of which no cooked food eater needs to contend with. My reference to **shock from a drastic diet change applies mainly to consistent *long-term* Raw Dieting.** Being Raw Vegan for one month, and then returning to cooked meat four times a week will not have very detrimental effects. If Raw Vegan 10-years, however, eating cooked meat again would create a considerable disturbance.

Eliminating cooked meat is a dietary improvement, but there are many more nutritional layers remaining. If I were eating the typical SAD diet, meat is the last thing I would eliminate. **The harm from refined sugar and processed starches is tenfold that of flesh food.** Please don't misunderstand me – a step forward in your diet is always a step forward! In terms of going backwards as this gentleman did however, small changes are small risk, and huge changes in diet need to be treated with more care.

2.   Why is it that my mom improved her diet, did a series of Colonic Irrigations, and the results were not as beneficial as I assumed they would be?

If your mom consistently eats a better diet by eliminating certain harmful foods from her diet *completely without any exceptions,* at some point she will go through a healing crisis. The best time for demonstrating the power of Colon Hydrotherapy is during a healing crisis. When she gets sick, when the doctors want to put her on antibiotics - that is when the results of Colon Hydrotherapy will be MIRACULOUS. **Otherwise, the effects of internal cleansing can sometimes be difficult to see, and thus difficult to appreciate.**

Time and time again I have heard the amusing stories of perplexed doctors prescribing antibiotics to patients who actually, after a series of Colonics, find they don't need a single pill.

All disease is the same – it is the accumulation of waste in the body. As the body struggles to expel this toxicity through the various eliminatory channels, familiar symptoms arise such as infection, rashes, acne, headaches, a runny nose, fatigue, as well as more obvious signs of imbalance such as bronchitis, strep throat, psoriasis, and eczema. Antibiotics are a common 'band-aid' for such symptoms. Often, however, even though they may offer temporary relief, **modern medical solutions throw the body into catastrophic imbalance. The monster of excess waste then starts growling and clawing inside of us, emerging later as a severe illness.**

3. Can Colon Hydrotherapy become an addiction?

Anything can become an addiction, including Colon Hydrotherapy. Some people over-exercise to compensate for their excessive eating habits. I call this "exercise bulimia". The same holds true with Colonic Irrigations. I find it incongruous to use Colon Hydrotherapy as a daily practice for long periods of time. **When Colonic Irrigation is used frequently to offset the effects of poor eating, I call this "colonic bulimia."**

I believe Colon Hydrotherapy is the most powerful cleansing tool a person can utilize. **People suffering from colonic bulimia unnaturally stimulate their healing to the next level.** They continually cleanse their colon, which purifies their bloodstream allowing the cells to release more and more endogenous poisons. This results in the contraction of the cells, bringing them to new levels of health and sensitivity. In cleaner states there is less margin for error, (inconsistencies in quality/quantity of food), and the body will demand an improved diet. **The problem is that these individuals are not usually improving**

their diet. Less-than-optimal eating habits produce excessive fermentative gas, which is exceedingly harmful to a cleaner body. Thus, they develop an ongoing reliance on using Colon Hydrotherapy every day for relief from the discomfort they otherwise feel. This abuse may catch up with them in the long-run.

It is stated in the book "Rebuild Your Health with Dr. Ann Wigmore's Living Foods Lifestyle":

> *I have heard people say that enemas are habit forming. I find this conception to be absurd. Considering the condition of the diseased colon, I cannot think of any better habit to have. Once the colon has been brought back to health, there is no longer such a great need for this systematic colon cleansing. Although, it should be stressed that keeping the colon healthy is a life-long process.*
>
> *(Rebuild Your Health with Dr. Ann Wigmore's Living Foods Lifestyle, Pg. 71)*

4.   Can someone develop a physical dependency on Colonic Irrigations? Does the colon lose muscle tone if it isn't being used? In other words: can we lose the ability to poop on our own?

I believe that an emotional dependency on Colonics may arise, but to directly answer the question: no, nothing suggests to me that Colon Hydrotherapy is physically weakening to any part of the body.

I have no documented paperwork to prove that frequent Colon Hydrotherapy does not cause atrophy of the colon muscle. What I do have, however, is personal experience and mass testimonial. Personally, there were stretches of time in my earlier years being Raw when I did Colonics *a couple of times a week,* and my elimination after those weeks was **better than ever.** Those I know who have done lengthy 2-3 month cleanses with daily colon treatments, report the same pattern. Bowel movements not only resume, but peristalsis and colon tone seem vastly improved.

To further answer the question, 'Do we lose the ability to poop on our own?'...that is actually one issue that Colonics can *remedy!* Constipation (the inability to poop on our own) is a common ailment among Americans. Coupled with a cleaner diet, Colon Hydrotherapy is the #1 aid for those suffering from constipation.

There is A LOT of waste inside of us. I know people who have lived on vegetable and fruit juices ONLY for well over three months. Enemas were part of the protocol during these juicing marathons. Each of these people reported that solid waste was being eliminated from their colon for the entire duration. That is three months of solids coming out of their bodies, without any solids actually being put *in!* I think this clearly demonstrates the amount of waste most people have inside them to release.

Instead of letting waste build up in their system, many enjoy cleansing their colon weekly with Enemas or Colonics. After a Colonic, bowel movements may not occur for 24 – 48 hours. That is OK, since the colon was completely cleaned out. The waste will build up once again, and you will resume your typical daily bowel movements.

As I said previously, although there is no physical dependency, one may experience *emotional* dependency. Once the colon is free from the years of excess waste that had embedded and hardened along its walls, you will likely experience the near-orgasmic joy of a clean colon. If someone practices Colon Hydrotherapy many times a week, they can become hooked on that clean, high vibration of an empty colon, and they will not enjoy coming down from that. **Although their bowels work perfectly, an emotional dependency can form.** They are unwilling to experience anything less than this level of cleanliness.

Others are fanatical about their level of body cleanliness, which is another type of emotional dependency. Toxins plague their system from nervous tension and other negative energies related to perfectionism. Additionally, in a nervous, contracted state, the body may have difficulty flowing, and in some cases peristalsis of the intestines may stop for a time. Many of you may experience this while traveling on planes and/or being in other people's homes – you just can't quite relax enough to poop. This can happen to anyone.

For stress-induced constipation, I recommend a magnesium supplement. The product *Natural Calm* is completely natural, and acts as a muscle relaxant. Its main ingredient is magnesium citrate. *Natural Calm* helps quiet the nerves and also facilitates sleeping for those suffering from insomnia or a restless night. Additionally, it assists bowel movements by relaxing us from our contracted state. *{You can find Natural Calm in the Resource Guide at the back of the book. Because it is helping so many people, many health food stores are also beginning to carry this product.}*

It is stated in the book "Rebuild Your Health with Dr. Ann Wigmore's Living Foods Lifestyle":

> *I have also heard people say that the colon becomes dependent on enema taking and will not work properly by itself. Again, the colon cannot possibly work when it is in such a toxic and diseased state. The colon will actually become less dependent on enemas as it becomes healthier through enemas and colonics and wheatgrass implants.*
>
> *(Rebuild Your Health with Dr. Ann Wigmore's Living Foods Lifestyle, Pg. 71)*

5.   Doesn't flushing the colon with water wash away our healthy bacteria?

There are two types of bacteria in the colon: (1) Beneficial and (2) Pathogenic. When the colon is compromised with waste – as it is for 95% of today's Americans – the pathogenic bacteria take over and destroy the beneficial bacteria. **Through Colon Cleansing, you create a clean, alkaline environment where beneficial bacteria can thrive and 'reclaim the land', so to speak.**

I have personally never had an issue with lack of beneficial bacteria in my colon. **Dr. Norman Walker lived well past the century mark and was a fiery advocate for frequent Colon Cleansing.** After a Colonic, he would drink a glass of carrot/spinach juice. This combination helped him "repopulate" the beneficial bacteria in the colon. These days we also have probiotics, for the same purpose.

6. Is there much difference between the salt water flush (as recommended in the Master Cleanse) and a Colonic? I personally have done the salt water flushes and have benefited greatly. But you speak so highly of Colonics that it makes me wonder if there is that big a difference between the two.

The reason the Master Cleanse is so beneficial is based on the principle of what you are not doing (refer to Appendix A, "What We Don't Eat"). You are Abstaining from all cooked and solid foods. In essence it is like going on a juice fast, with maple syrup thrown in. The simple fact that you are leaving all those other foods out and only having those liquids means you will start healing. Another benefit that happens when someone does a salt flush is that it empties the bowels. This can provide a tremendous relief.

You can use salt water flushes if you like, yet if you are truly on the life-long fast of being 100% raw, it is highly recommended that you do Colonic Irrigations once a month for optimal long-term success. Would you rather fast 10 days a month doing the salt water flush or would you rather simply walk in and have a Colonic Irrigation done in an hour, or even do it with alternative methods right in your own home? Additionally, if you are truly 100% Raw, at some point the maple syrup may affect you – you may feel low energy and it would be less than optimal for your health.

7. How would you define Detoxification?

Detoxification can be defined as endogenous ma-

terial (waste matter inside a cell) leaving the cell and entering our blood stream, eventually exiting the body via the lungs, skin, kidneys, or large intestine. This release of stored toxins from the cell is **triggered when the intake of that harmful substance is stopped.** For example, if a drug addict eliminated cocaine, they would go through withdrawal, a definite symptom of detoxification. The same holds true with our food intake. **If a cooked food eater completely eliminates processed starches from their diet, they too will experience withdrawal/ detoxification.**

8. Why is it that I don't feel good after a Colonic?

On occasion, a person may not feel well after Colonic Irrigation. When you cleanse the colon thoroughly with water, all the waste and gas pressure is removed. With this vast 'extra' space in the colon, the organs and cells now have the chance to eliminate the accumulated toxins within their structure, causing a purging of waste throughout the system. It's like having a kitchen sink full of sludge, and then removing the stopper or plug – everything is going to empty from the sink (our body) into the pipes below (our colon). Generally, this is one of the reasons why a series of Colonic Irrigations is recommended.

9. Can a person become too clean?

It depends on what a person is trying to accomplish. Often I've found that the reason people want to refine their health is because **the cleaner we are, the more**

our body becomes in-tune and receptive to spiritual energy. The amount of vibrational energy being channeled through my Raw body now, compared to when I was a cooked food eater, is astronomical. Mainstream thinkers seem to find my stories crazy and people who knew me before I went Raw see me as a completely different person.

If a Raw Foodist eliminates certain concentrated foods such as nuts, or transitions to a Fruitarian, Liquidarian or Breatharian lifestyle, they will become even more sensitive. These **extremes can affect their long-term success.** At first, they may feel increasingly strong and vital. However, in the long-run they would not be able to endure the adverse environmental conditions facing our planet today. **Some people may prefer a highly spiritual life to a long life.** Even though I fervently aim for both, I don't intend risking going past the 100% Raw Vegan stage of 'cleanliness'.

10. What is your favorite Raw Food? How often do you eat it?

I have many favorite Raw Foods. TOP Favorites ...*avocados, durian, and figs,* also nuts and seeds (in moderate quantities). I love drinking all sorts of vegetable juice combinations. **Mixing carrot juice with greens, especially spinach – it's like my coffee, gotta have it!**

11. What is true hunger? How long does it take the average human to experience true hunger after eating?

Hunger is generally defined as a strong desire or

"need" for food. Detoxification begins when there is an absence of food, and feelings of detox are often mistaken for hunger. If you are consistently eating three times a day, you will experience "hunger" three times a day. If you were to eat only twice, your body would go through withdrawal, as it starts to detox. People just assume this means they are hungry, and they eat. There are numerous documented cases, and even more undocumented, of people fasting on only water for 30 days and beyond. Obviously then, the feelings of hunger we typically experience are not necessarily SOS signals for food needed to sustain life. Hunger rarely means, "Eat NOW or Die!" **I define hunger as the regulator of detoxification.**

12. Have you changed any of your eating habits since becoming a Raw Vegan? Like: more of one thing, less of another?

If one truly adheres to a 100% Raw Vegan Diet, they will evolve into needing less and less food. When I first started, I would eat three large avocados in one meal and a few pounds of fruit. These days I only eat about one avocado per day, and rarely eat over a pound of fruit, ever. In the future, I can see these quantities reducing as well.

13. Tell us one of the most interesting Raw success stories that you have heard.

A man had AIDS. Through persistence and expert guidance on cleansing and the Raw Diet, the AIDS be came undetectable in medical testing. **Raw Food is not a cure-all, but I have seen "miracles" take place.**

14. What, in your opinion, is one of the largest negative side effects of the Raw Food Diet?

For me, the spiritual rewards far surpass any negative effects that one may experience as a Raw Foodist. Personally, I was most challenged by the confusion my body experienced, from my overnight transition to Raw Foods. It took a while to balance out and settle into the new way of eating. **Patience and consistency are highly beneficial for this tremendous journey.**

APPENDIX C
COLONIC IRRIGATION TESTIMONIALS

Colon Hydrotherapy is Miraculous! I can almost guarantee literal miracles taking place in your body, should you choose Colonic Irrigation. Below are just a few examples of lives that were changed:

Before my lecture at a health food store in Ohio, a man came up asking for guidance. He was set against Colonics, convinced he was squeaky clean and had no need for internal irrigation. He sat through my entire talk and then left. About two weeks later, I received an email from him:

I am down to 150 lbs and cannot believe how much better I look and feel!!! The colonic did it!!! My skin is so much clearer, my hair is fuller and thicker, and it sure looks to me like there is more of it. Thanks again for your advice, and I will also continue on E3Live® several days a week.

The next week he emailed me again reporting:

Since I did that colonic last week, I have lost another 5 lbs! My stomach is flat, and I no longer crave sugar, bread, or salt. I even have to go out and buy new clothing. I am eating more salads, but can you recommend anything else to keep my digestion and colon clean? I have not tried any probiotics since my diet is vegan, and about 95% organic.

Seven months later, this gentleman contacted me again:

As you may recall from our last correspondence, I had a colonic 7 months ago and promptly lost about 15 lbs. Five of those pounds have returned. The colonic I had last summer really helped, but I am not sure if I really need another. Is there some kind of home-based colon cleanse that I can do? I have heard organic cayenne powder and organic olive oil, along with organic lemon works.

I am starting to feel somewhat sluggish and a little more tired than usual. Right now I do not think I need anything as extreme as a colonic, but I remember how much the one I had earlier helped. Do you think one is needed? Please let me know.

Of course, my advice was another Colonic. I also gave him the option of an at-home Colema Board® or 6-quart Enema Bag. Although not as effective as a professionally administered colonic, they get the job done. To avoid dealing with the learning curve, and because he had been uncomfortable for some time, I told him to just go get a Colonic and look into purchasing another tool for at-home use. The large Enema Bag and Colema Board® are ideal and financially savvy options for people who want to cleanse their colon more than three times a year.

Here were his results:

I cannot believe the changes in just one day. My skin, digestion, appetite, breathing!! Everything is better after just one colonic.

So much came out of my system. It seemed like a dead rat was stuck inside my colon and intestines. Even my urine is clear now. I would recommend a colonic to everyone at least twice a year. It works!!! It gets so much junk out of your system and improves your digestion. It is now mandatory for me.

Thanks again for the advice and help. I will try to do another in about 3-6 months and continue to watch my diet.

Below I have included my correspondence with another younger man, and his results with Colonic Irrigation.

Hey Matt,

I am a 19-year-old college student in Boston, MA, and I became 100% Raw in November 2006 because of a strong desire to live as long and as vitally as I possibly can. With the exception of a few meals here and there (out of peer pressure, cravings, etc. in college) I have maintained pure Raw consumption.

Physically, I have felt amazing, and honestly could never see myself eating any other way for the rest of my life. When I consume cooked foods, I get clear signals from my body that I should avoid them. Although my physical health has been incredible, my mental health has been questionable; I have been severely depressed on a number of occasions since going Raw.

I was wondering if this might have had to do with my being in a cold environment as a 100% Raw Vegan (Boston winter in December is below 0!) or potential effects from water fasting during a time of mental stress (pre-finals). I had heard wonderful things about water fasting (I read a lot of books by Daniel Reid, and they were my catalyst for going Raw, fasting, etc.) Lots of info,

I know, but it's so uplifting and inspiring to see that there are others out there like myself.

If you have any responses to the correlation between mental health and becoming Raw, I'd love to hear them. I can't wait to read your book, and hope we can develop some sort of relationship, as you seem like a really interesting guy. I also love yoga (Bikram particularly) and would love to share experiences/advice/etc. about any and all subjects if you're up for it. Hope to hear from you!

Sincerely,
Mark

When detoxification happens these poisons travel through our blood stream and can start to have an effect on our mental health. I told Mark that a series of Colonic Irrigations would be invaluable to him.

Matt,
Thanks so much for the advice. The Colonics are working wonders, you were so right. We have a Colema Board® and it's awesome.

I read your book in one night, actually, as you did with that other book pre-Raw Veganism. Although my sensitivity to toxins will increase from being all Raw, I'm ready and willing to experience life to the fullest. I already feel much better from eating 100% for a mere 2 weeks, without any cheating.

Anyway, I'm sure you're really busy being a Raw Food pioneer, but I just wanted to say thanks for taking the time to respond to my question. Hope all's well, hopefully I'll speak with you soon,
Mark

From another gentlemen new to Colonics:

Matt,

The colonic really made a difference. I am again eating more greens and fruits, walking more and GROWING MORE HAIR!!!! My skin has cleared up and I am alternating steam-distilled water with some spring and well water.

Recently, a female customer from my website wrote me:

Thanks! I am looking forward to my occasional Raw treats that I ordered.

After reading your book and listening to you talk in Charlotte, I decided I didn't want my diet to become too pure. I don't want to become too sensitive. I have been 6 weeks Raw and I agree with you, the Colonics make all the difference!

Lastly, a great friend of mine recently improved her diet and had a Colonic Irrigation:

Just had my first colonic it was great! Didn't have much matter, mostly gas. I was so bloated and feeling really sluggish. Now I feel great you were right. Thanks again Matt!!!!!!!!!!!!!!!!!!!!!
Rose

Remember, it is the GAS – detoxification from our cells – that we want to exit the body. Review the section "The Science Behind It All" for more on gases.

RESOURCES

The following resources, except one, can be ordered from:

www.TheRawFoodWorld.com

6-quart Enema Bag – The colon holds between 4-6 quarts. This Enema Bag is a valuable resource for cleansing and is ideal for traveling.

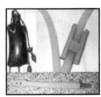

Colema Board® – The Colema Board® is a gravity method Colon Cleansing system that you can do from home. Five gallons of water allows for multiple fills and releases.

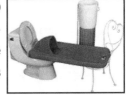

B12, B6, and Folic Acid – I have found this B-vitamin supplement to be the best on the market. Blood tests reveal my B12 levels are healthy. The pill does contain trace amounts of fructose. I could probably consume the entire bottle without any adverse effects. If I can handle it, I feel fine recommending it to others. Dr. Fred Bisci, 40-year Raw Vegan, also takes this product, without any problem.

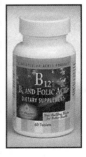

OceanGrown Seawater Solution – Pure and clean seawater derived from the Florida oceans. It provides 59 Trace Elements. Add a few drops to Vegetable Juice, Fruit Juice, and water to re-

1 Quart Twin Neck

ceive the benefits. At this point, the manufacturer only recommends it for growing vegetation. However, I feel there is great advantage derived from also adding it to the liquids I drink.

Angstrom Minerals Zinc – Zinc is the only element needed for every single function of our body. I take Zinc in angstrom form to ensure best absorption.

Norwalk Juicer – Designed by Dr. Norman Walker, this machine costs over $2,000. I feel the benefits are well worth the money. The triturating action opens every cell of the vegetation and the hydraulic press then squeezes out maximum nutrition from the fibers. The nutrient quality of juice from the Norwalk is unsurpassed. Kept in the refrigerator, the juice remains vital for up to three days. Available from: www.NorwalkJuicers.com

Green Star Juicer – Another great juicer with high nutrient quality. This twin-gear model squeezes the juice out of the vegetables without heating even the most fibrous greens.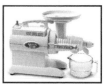

Dr Fred Bisci's Therapeutic Enzyme Blend – The most powerful enzyme blend on the market. Their power is undeniable.

Natural Calm – Natural Calm is a completely natural formula that acts as a muscle relaxant. The main ingredient is magnesium citrate. Natural Calm helps quiet the nerves and also facilitates sleeping for those suffering from insomnia or a restless night. Additionally, it assists bowel movements by relaxing us from any stressful, contracted state.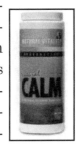

Nut Milk Bags – Great for straining vegetable juice, growing sprouts and making nut milks.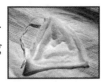

Dr Norman Walker's Books – We carry the entire collection of Dr. Norman Walker books and charts. Enjoy them all!
Become Younger
The Vegetarian Guide to Diet & Salad
Fresh Vegetable and Fruit Juices
Natural Way to Vibrant Health
Water Can Undermine Your Health
Colon Health
Weight Control, Pure & Simple
Colon Therapy Chart
Foot Relaxation Chart
Endocrine Glands Chart

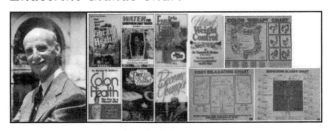

Other recommended books referenced in
Raw Success:

Raw Food and Health, by St. Louis Estes
Man's Higher Consciousness, by Hilton Hotema

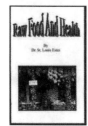 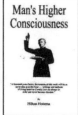

***The above resources, except one, can be ordered
from:***
<u>**www.TheRawFoodWorld.com**</u>

NOTES

NOTES

NOTES

NOTES